'I Wish I Hadn't Eaten That'

Simple Dietary Solutions
for the 20 Most Common
Health Problems

Maria Cross

HAY HOUSE

Australia • Canada • Hong Kong • India
South Africa • United Kingdom • United States

First published and ... Kingdom by:
Hay House U ... London W ... ... (44) 20 8962 1230;
Fax: (44) ... www.hayhouse ...

Published and distributed in the United States of America by:
Ha ... ... Suite 100, Carlsbad, CA ...
Tel.: (1) 760 431 7695 or (800) ... Fax: (1) 760 431 6948 or (800) 650 5115.
www.hayhouse ...

Published and distributed in Australia by:
Hay House Australia Ltd, 18/36 Ralph St, Alexandria NSW 2015. Tel.: (61) 2 9669 4299;
Fax: (61) 2 9669 4144. www.hayhouse.com.au

Published and distributed in the Republic of South Africa by:
Hay House SA (Pty), Ltd, PO Box 990, Witkoppen 2068. Tel./Fax: (27) 11 467 8904.
www.hayhouse.co.za

Published and distributed in India by:
Hay House Publishers India, Muskaan Complex, Plot No.3, B-2, Vasant Kunj, New Delhi – 110
070. Tel.: (91) 11 4176 1620; Fax: (91) 11 4176 1630. www.hayhouse.co.in

Distributed in Canada by:
Raincoast, 9050 Shaughnessy St, Vancouver, BC V6P 6E5. Tel.: (1) 604 323 7100;
Fax: (1) 604 323 2600

© Maria Cross, 2011

The moral rights of the author have been asserted.

The information given in this book should not be treated as a substitute for professional medical
advice; always consult a medical practitioner. Any use of the information in this book is at the
reader's discretion and risk. Neither the author nor the publisher can be held responsible for any
loss, claim or damage arising out of the use, or misuse, or the suggestions made or the failure to
take medical advice.

A catalogue record for this book is available from the British Library.

ISBN 978-1-84850-374-8

Printed and bound in the UK by
CPI Mackays, Chatham ME5 8TD

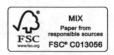

For Peter

Contents

Introduction

Everyone's a nutrition expert nowadays. Whatever your health problem you'll find a legion of pundits lining up to tell you what to eat – from your mother, partner and work colleague to celebrity chefs on TV. Every newspaper, whatever its persuasion or profundity, is determined to give you the best, most current advice on the latest meal-time trend. Watching the dressing-down of the obese and benighted for their dietary misdemeanours on prime-time TV has become a national sport. There's so much nutrition information available now that half the country can talk eloquently of the role of friendly bacteria and omega-3 fatty acids, or the crucial need for antioxidants to combat free radicals. Yet it wasn't that long ago that we barely knew a vitamin from a mineral, or a protein from a carbohydrate.

This modern dietary enlightenment is a good thing. We are becoming increasingly aware, for example, that feeding children a diet of junk food can transform them into manic monsters. That what we eat and drink can have a profound effect on mood, and that we shouldn't necessarily believe everything that food manufacturers would have us believe. Our recently acquired nutritional nous has steered us away from blind faith in official pronouncements of safety and wholesomeness towards an intuitive awareness of what is good and right to eat and what is decidedly questionable.

This increased awareness has come about at a time when the British palate has, thankfully, become more sophisticated and started demanding better quality food. No longer the laughing stock of food fashionistas, British food is deeply trendy these days. So too is nostalgia for home cooking. Once, the notion of cooking real food was parodied by adverts such as the Martian 'Smash' men, hooting deliriously at the idea of anyone actually taking the time to boil a pan of spuds. Now we can't get enough home cooking, or we at least lament the hectic lifestyles which restrict quality kitchen-time. And if you lack the skills, you can learn from TV chefs who tempt the goddess within us all to return to home baking and simple culinary pleasures.

With the state of the nation's health, a transition from 'gruel Britannia' to traditional quality fare may be just the medicine we need. For the majority of people, however, interest in good food is yet to be translated into healthy eating habits. A quarter of adults are now classified as obese, and whatever it is they are eating it certainly isn't fresh fruit and vegetables. The latest national diet and nutrition survey reported that in 2008/9 only 33 per cent of women and 37 per cent of men participating in the survey were meeting the 'five-a-day' guidelines. Worse still, only 7 per cent of girls and 22 per cent of boys aged 11 to 18 were doing so.

There are many other people who may not be obese but who are still not achieving optimum health with a sense of total wellbeing. They might not have rampant heart disease, diabetes or cancer, or any other chronic disease currently terrorizing the Western world, but they are still simply *not well*. They may have an intuitive understanding that diet is in some way part of the problem, but the link between illness and nutrition remains elusive.

I have been practising as a nutritional therapist since 1994, advising clients on a variety of health problems. I see the same problems over and over again, and very rarely am I unable to help those clients eliminate or greatly reduce their symptoms. Most of these people are not seriously ill, but their symptoms are debilitating enough to make them feel, at times, quite wretched. I have come to identify 20 common symptoms which people complain of most frequently. They are:

1. lack of energy ('tired all the time' is the most common complaint I hear)

2. weight gain

3. constipation

4. diarrhoea

5. bloating and/or flatulence

6. frequent colds/infections

7. aching joints

8. mild depression and/or anxiety

9. dry skin and/or eyes

10. headaches

11. acne

12. food cravings

13. poor circulation

14. insomnia

15. poor memory and/or concentration

16. mood swings

17. premenstrual syndrome

18. period pain

19. skin rashes, itching, eruptions, etc.

20. water retention.

I sometimes think of my clients as the walking wounded. More often than not, they look fine enough. Indeed, they don't usually have any diagnosed medical condition as such. They hold down jobs – sometimes very important ones at that – and bring up children whilst running busy households. Their juggling skills are heroic. Most – but by no means all – of my clients are women and their narratives reveal extraordinary multi-tasking skills. But hardy as they appear, inside they are struggling with exhaustion, stress and anxiety about their health.

Because of my experience, I am convinced that there are very few truly 'healthy' people. Most people appear to be functioning below par, and have just learned to adapt their lives to cope with at least one of the above 20 symptoms. This book is intended for all those of you who are perfectly healthy but not very well; who have had a raft of tests all confirming your good health, contrary to the way you actually feel; those of you who know that your health is not what it could and should be, but are frustrated when you try to find answers in conventional places.

This is what a typical, fed-up client will say to me:

'I've seen my GP. He's done all the tests and says there is nothing wrong with me. I'm not going back because he thinks I'm making it up and just wants to put me on antidepressants.'

It is frustrating to have to soldier on with health problems without knowing why you've got them, or what to do about them. This frustration is not all bad, however, when it engenders a determination to take control of your own health and get to the root of the matter. The result can be enlightening and uplifting, and often involves complementary therapy.

Nutritional therapy can be extraordinarily effective. It does require effort; the client does all the work, based upon recommendations made. But the pay-off for this approach is empowerment for the client, not to mention results.

Nutrition is not the answer to every health problem, because nothing in life is ever that simple. But it is the cornerstone of good health, and should always be the starting point on the road to total wellbeing. A good nutritional therapist will look at the patient's collection of symptoms, cross-reference with his or her diet and lifestyle and join up the dots. This book is designed to help you take this same approach in order to achieve a long-term, effective solution to those persistent health problems which, like background noise, just won't go away.

This book will help you identify the underlying dietary *origins* of your particular cluster of symptoms and work on those origins through nutritional means. It is utterly pointless to look for remedies for symptoms without first identifying the reasons they arose. Many complementary practitioners are quick to criticize conventional doctors for hastily writing out prescriptions without addressing the cause of a patient's condition, yet blithely do something very similar themselves. Taking vitamins or minerals, herbal and other remedies to deal with a particular symptom is the same thing as swallowing a drug and waiting for the symptom to vanish. Once you stop taking the drug, or the remedy, the problem is likely to reappear, because its underlying cause has not been identified or addressed. Working on the origin of a problem, rather than just treating the symptoms, is absolutely fundamental to re-establishing health and equilibrium on a long-term basis.

Dealing with the same symptoms over and over meant that, in time, I came to identify the most likely diet-related causes of those symptoms. Each chapter of this book (apart from the Meal Ideas chapter) is devoted to one of those causes. I have outlined exactly what I as a nutritional therapist would do if you were my client suffering from one or more of the 'top 20' symptoms. I will guide you to making the right dietary changes for you by first identifying the underlying factors affecting your health, and then working out how you need to adapt your diet to have a therapeutic effect – that is, to eliminate or reduce your symptoms. I may suggest tests you can have carried out privately, or supplements which can help boost the effects of dietary change.

There are times when nutrition works well in conjunction with other therapies, such as herbalism, acupuncture or reflexology. In this book I will state when I think it is appropriate to consider other therapies alongside nutrition, for a more holistic approach. *All the advice given in this book is based on the assumption that you have already seen your GP and advised him or her of your health issues, and are currently taking no medication.*

A WORD ON NUTRITIONAL THERAPY

You will have noticed that I used the term 'nutritional therapist' and not 'nutritionist' or 'dietitian'. Although many people use these terms interchangeably, there is a difference between each profession. A dietitian is currently the only nutrition professional regulated by law, and whose title is also protected by law. He or she holds either a four-year degree in dietetics, or a science degree followed by a two-year postgraduate qualification. Most dietitians work within the NHS, either in a hospital setting or an outpatient department. They may work in general wards or in intensive care, where special feeding, such as tube-feeding, is required. Some choose to specialize in one area, such as paediatrics. To see an NHS dietitian as an outpatient requires a GP referral, though some practitioners do work as consultants in private practice. A dietitian will give dietary advice to people suffering from a chronic disease such as obesity or diabetes. They may also advise parents of children who are failing to thrive.

The term 'nutritionist' is not currently protected by law, and for this reason it is often used to describe anyone who knows anything about nutrition. The problem here is that any unqualified person can call him- or herself a nutritionist, or indeed – for effect – clinical nutritionist. The Nutrition Society (which describes itself as a learned society whose aim is to 'advance the scientific study of nutrition and its application to the maintenance of human and animal health') has defined 'nutritionist' as a scientist working in a particular field such as the food industry or the media. Most of the large supermarket chains employ in-house nutritionists to communicate positive messages about their products. Public health nutritionists work in communities to promote health, or get involved in policy development or campaign work. In as far as the Nutrition Society has defined the role, nutritionists do not give direct diet advice to individuals, as they are not trained in clinical practice.

Nutritional therapists such as myself, on the other hand, *are* trained in clinical practice. Having said that, as the law currently stands anyone can still call themselves a nutritional therapist whatever their level of training. Thankfully that is soon likely to change, as nutritional therapy is a profession undergoing rapid transformation and currently pursuing statutory regulation. The overwhelming majority of nutritional therapists are glad of this. The therapy's regulatory body is the Complementary and Natural

Healthcare Council, and all training schools must meet standards set down in the National Occupational Standards produced by the Skills for Business network. In 1999 the University of Westminster launched the first degree course in nutritional therapy, setting the standard for the profession overall.

The main difference between dietitians and nutritional therapists is that the latter, who work largely in private practice, have a greater focus on individual dietary requirements and believe that dietary changes can have a therapeutic effect. Personalized diets and the judicious use of food supplements are recommended to help achieve optimal health. Nutritional therapists focus on the link between health and diet, with an emphasis on identifying the dietary triggers of a health problem. This is achieved by examining the client's context: family history of illness, lifestyle, exercise regime, exposure to toxins (as in, for example, dental amalgams) and medical history, such as use of antibiotics and other pharmaceuticals. The professional body to which accredited practitioners belong is the British Association of Applied Nutrition and Nutritional Therapy (BANT). See BANT's details in Resources if you wish to find an accredited therapist in your area.

How to Use This Book

Discovering the cause of your symptoms is a crucial first step on the path to wellness. A bit of detective work is required here, but if you follow the guide below you should be able to identify the reasons for your symptoms, so that you can then address them.

Start by studying the table below. In the left-hand column I have listed the most common symptoms experienced by the 'perfectly healthy but not very well'. In the middle column are listed the most likely dietary origins of those symptoms, from a nutritional therapy perspective, and column three tells you which chapter you need to focus on.

Symptom	Possible diet-related cause	Solution/ chapter
Aching joints	Food intolerance	1
	Fatty acid deficiency	4
	Leaky gut syndrome	8
Acne	Food intolerance	1
	Blood-sugar imbalance	2
	Fatty acid deficiency	4
	Oestrogen dominance	5
	Dysbiosis	7
	Leaky gut syndrome	8

Symptom	Possible diet-related cause	Solution/chapter
Bloating and/or flatulence	Food intolerance	1
	Blood-sugar imbalance	2
	Dysbiosis	7
	Leaky gut syndrome	8
Circulation – poor	Mild hypothyroidism	6
Colds/infections – frequent	Food intolerance	1
	Blood-sugar imbalance	2
	Adrenal fatigue	3
	Dysbiosis	7
Constipation	Food intolerance	1
	Mild hypothyroidism	6
	Dysbiosis	7
	Leaky gut syndrome	8
Cravings	Food intolerance	1
	Blood-sugar imbalance	2
	Adrenal fatigue	3
Depression and/or anxiety	Food intolerance	1
	Blood-sugar imbalance	2
	Adrenal fatigue	3
	Fatty acid deficiency	4
	Oestrogen dominance	5
	Mild hypothyroidism	6
	Leaky gut syndrome	8
Diarrhoea	Food intolerance	1
	Dysbiosis	7
	Leaky gut syndrome	8
Dry skin and/or eyes	Fatty acid deficiency	4

Symptom	Possible diet-related cause	Solution/chapter
Fatigue	Food intolerance	1
	Blood-sugar imbalance	2
	Adrenal fatigue	3
	Fatty acid deficiency	4
	Mild hypothyroidism	6
	Dysbiosis	7
	Leaky gut syndrome	8
Headache	Food intolerance	1
	Blood-sugar imbalance	2
	Adrenal fatigue	3
	Oestrogen dominance	5
	Leaky gut syndrome	8
Insomnia	Food intolerance	1
	Blood-sugar imbalance	2
	Adrenal fatigue	3
Memory/ concentration – poor	Food intolerance	1
	Blood-sugar imbalance	2
	Adrenal fatigue	3
	Fatty acid deficiency	4
	Mild hypothyroidism	6
	Leaky gut syndrome	8
Mood swings	Food intolerance	1
	Blood-sugar imbalance	2
	Adrenal fatigue	3
	Essential fatty acid deficiency	4
	Oestrogen dominance	5
Period pain	Essential fatty acid deficiency	4
Premenstrual syndrome	Blood-sugar imbalance	2
	Essential fatty acid deficiency	4
	Oestrogen dominance	5

Symptom	Possible diet-related cause	Solution/chapter
Skin rashes, itching, eruptions, etc.	Food intolerance	1
	Blood-sugar imbalance	2
	Fatty acid deficiency	4
	Dysbiosis	7
	Leaky gut syndrome	8
Water retention	Food intolerance	1
	Oestrogen dominance	5
	Mild hypothyroidism	6
Weight gain (inexplicable)	Food intolerance	1
	Oestrogen dominance	5
	Mild hypothyroidism	6

Symptoms can be as complex and as elaborate as the human body itself, so I would never suggest that this table of possible causes is exhaustive. But as far as dietary investigations go, it's pretty comprehensive.

As you can see, deciding where to start can be straightforward, but often isn't. For example, if your one and only symptom is period pain, then you can go straight to Solution 4 (page 59) and read about the link between fatty acid deficiency, pain and inflammation. However, if you suffer from acne or fatigue, for example, there are quite a few possible dietary links, in which case you will need to work out which is the most likely culprit and start with that one.

How do you do that? This is best explained by example. Let's look at 'Mary', who is fictitious but whose symptoms are fairly typical. In the left-hand column is a list of her symptoms, and in the right-hand column are the relevant chapters which she should read.

Example 1 – Mary's Symptoms

symptom	relevant solution/chapter
fatigue	1,**2**,3,4,6,7,8
anxiety	1,**2**,3,4,5,6,8
mood swings	1,**2**,3,4,5
PMS	**2**,4,5
cravings	1,**2**,3

As you can see, the one common denominator of all these symptoms is the subject of the chapter on Solution 2: blood-sugar imbalance. Therefore Mary should go straight to that chapter and follow the advice given there.

It is possible that once she has done so, all her symptoms will clear up, but let's assume that even after sorting out her blood-sugar imbalance she still has PMS. She should therefore turn her attention to the chapters addressing oestrogen dominance and fatty acid deficiency and follow the advice there.

Whenever there are digestive symptoms present, these should in most cases be addressed first, because digestive health is absolutely fundamental to overall health. Let's look at 'John'. John is not overweight or particularly stressed. He does, however, have a few digestive symptoms which have defied medical diagnosis. As with all mysterious digestive problems, I recommend eliminating the possibility of food intolerances first. The reason for this is that intolerance is such a common cause of gastrointestinal disturbance, and is also relatively quick and easy to determine, compared to other possibilities. Therefore John should read the Solution 1 chapter first – especially because, as you can see, food intolerance could be the underlying factor in all his symptoms. If indeed he does find that he has food intolerance, but, after eliminating the offending food still has one or two remaining symptoms, he should also read and act on the subjects of chapters 7 and 8, as these also feature prominently – and both directly affect the digestive system.

Example 2 – John's Symptoms

symptom	relevant solution/chapter
bloating	**1,2,7,8**
flatulence	**1,2,7,8**
constipation	**1,6,7,8**
occasional diarrhoea	**1,7,8**
insomnia	**1,2,3**
aching joints	**1,4,8**

You should by now have a clear idea of how nutritional therapy can work for you. I cannot stress enough, however, that you should first discuss your symptoms with your GP to make sure that you do not have an underlying medical condition which cannot and should not be addressed by food and diet alone. If you do not have any such medical condition, then there is, in my view, an extremely good chance that nutritional therapy may be just what you need.

Bear in mind also that some medications interact with some dietary supplements, so the advice in this book is only intended for people who are not taking any prescribed medications – in other words, the perfectly healthy but not very well.

Finally, once you have worked out what aspect of your diet is related to your health problems, you'll want to know what you can eat. The last chapter of this book provides meal ideas to help you make the right food choices for your individual needs.

Solution 1

Identifying Food Intolerances

Food intolerance is a likely culprit in almost every scenario. Also known as food sensitivity, food intolerance is both commonplace and extraordinarily diverse in terms of the possible symptoms it can cause. These symptoms often assume a chameleon-like quality, changing apparently at whim: one day a headache, another day a bloated stomach. To compound matters, the effects of unwittingly consuming something tasty yet pernicious often do not make themselves known for several days, making the culprit hard to isolate. No wonder that so few people ever ascertain the real cause of their niggling health problems. Instead, they just learn to live with them, having taken antibiotics, steroids and other pills, or rubbed in all sorts of creams, to no avail.

COMMON SYMPTOMS

If food intolerance is indeed the root of your problem, your symptoms are likely to be one or more of those listed on pages xv–xviii. In addition, you might also experience asthma and nasal congestion, or even hyperactivity.

We are all, of course, unique in our biochemical make-up, so the list is by no means exhaustive, but it does cover the most common reactions to a problem food. Sensitivities can affect every system of the body, and many people are astonished to find that something they eat can actually make them feel depressed, or bring on their asthma. Almost every possible digestive symptom you can think of can be attributed to a food intolerance, from constipation to diarrhoea (and back again), to bloating, flatulence and pain.

Having outlined the elusive nature of food intolerance, I would hasten to add that identifying the offender is relatively easy, once you know how. I therefore recommend you invest some energy into considering this area before researching other possibilities. Another reason you should think seriously about incriminating something you've eaten is that the whole area of intolerance is frequently dismissed, overlooked and ignored by conventional medicine, so chances are that if you do have a food sensitivity, nobody's noticed.

FURTHER CAUSES FOR SUSPICION

There is good reason to suspect a food intolerance if:

- you have at least one of the symptoms listed on pages xv–xviii which has so far evaded medical explanation

- symptoms come and go, inexplicably

- you crave certain foods.

This last point is especially telling. It is cruelly ironic that you quite possibly crave the foods which are compromising your health. It's often the very foods we love, and eat too much of for our own good, which turn out to be culpable. It's a bit like being addicted to a harmful substance, such as tobacco. It's bad for you but you want more. Bear in mind also that an intolerance can develop at any age; you can indulge your love of a particular food with impunity for years, then suddenly develop an intolerance just by dint of overdoing it.

NAME THAT REACTION

It is important to understand that there is a difference between food allergy and food intolerance. If you have an allergy to a particular food – known as an allergen – you probably already know about it. The reaction you experience from consuming an allergen is usually immediate and unquestionably caused by the food in question. Typically, a rash, swollen lips or tongue or headache may occur. True allergies are rare: fewer than 5 per cent of the population are believed to be affected. In severe cases, an allergic reaction can cause anaphylactic shock, an extreme reaction to a food (peanuts, dairy or shellfish in many cases) whereby the individual experiences difficulty breathing or speaking, dizziness and collapse, due to sudden loss of blood pressure. In such situations, immediate medical intervention is critical, as there is a real threat to life.

The allergic reaction is caused by the allergen triggering an immune system response. The body's immune system, in order to fight what it mistakenly perceives to be a threat, releases immunoglobulin E (IgE) antibodies. The production of these IgE antibodies results in the release of chemicals such as histamine, which give rise to the allergic response.

Allergies often run in families (which are thus known as 'atopic families'). Typical atopic allergic reactions include eczema, hay fever, rhinitis and asthma. The gene for an atopic allergy is passed from parent to child, though not all children will inherit the gene in question.

DIAGNOSING AN ALLERGY

If you suspect an allergy and would like to have it confirmed, you should consult your GP about testing. There are two tests you can have: a skin prick test or a blood test. The skin prick test involves scratching the skin and then applying a dilute solution containing extract of a suspected food (the allergen) to the skin. If you have a true allergy to that food, a reaction will occur within a few minutes – an itchy red rash or red bump will appear. The blood test, known as a RAST (radioallergosorbent test), measures levels of IgE antibodies in the blood for specific foods. The results are conclusive, even though your own experience of ingesting a particular allergen will probably have told you the same thing.

DEFINING INTOLERANCE

The fiendish intolerance is different. Its slippery, evasive nature makes it less identifiable. Perhaps it is because intolerances don't behave in a neat, orderly fashion that medics tend to downplay their significance. Traditionally, science has it that intolerance is rare and does not induce an immune response, and therefore you cannot test for an intolerance in the same way you can an allergy. Some nutritional heretics claim that that is simply not true – that the human body does indeed create antibodies to foods which create an intolerance reaction, and that those antibodies, and therefore foods, can be identified by blood tests. However, instead of stimulating the production of IgE antibodies, a food intolerance stimulates a different type of antibody: IgG. The production of IgG antibodies is slow, however, so the reaction to the offending item is delayed, by anything from a couple of hours to a few days.

The evidence that a food intolerance does stimulate an identifiable immune response is increasingly convincing but still highly controversial. In 2004 the medical journal *Gut* reported a randomized controlled trial of patients with irritable bowel syndrome which found that those who avoided foods to which they were found to have IgG antibodies were significantly more likely to have a reduction in symptoms than those who did not avoid IgG-positive foods.[1] The authors concluded that 'Food elimination based on IgG antibodies may be effective in reducing IBS symptoms and is worthy of further biomedical research.' That biomedical research has been ongoing and suspicions have continued. In 2005 an editorial in the *American Journal of Gastroenterology* suggested, in relation to IgG-mediated food intolerance in irritable bowel syndrome, that 'perhaps now is the time to revisit some of the immunological reactions to dietary antigens that, in the past, have been dismissed as irrelevant'.[2] Indeed, when researchers did just that, in 2007, they found that, of 5,286 patients who reported a wide range of chronic medical conditions, and who had taken a food-specific IgG blood test, 76 per cent experienced a notable improvement in their symptoms when they eliminated the foods to which they tested positive.[3]

Experts can be a strange lot and it is extremely difficult to say for sure just how many people are food-sensitive. Food intolerance expert Dr James Braly estimates that up to 50 per cent of people have an unknown food sensitivity.[4] The British Nutrition Foundation (largely funded by the food industry), on the other hand, claims that only 1 to 2 per cent of the population can claim a genuine food intolerance, with many others – 20 per cent of people – only imagining such an affliction.[5]

My experience as a nutritional therapist compels me to believe that the truth lies somewhere in between. Whatever the true figure, the fact is that I consistently find that, once a suspect item is removed from a client's daily diet, long-standing health problems clear up almost immediately.

FOODS MOST LIKELY TO CAUSE A REACTION

It is usually a protein within a food which is responsible for any adverse reaction. For this reason, many people who are sensitive to dairy foods are fine with butter, which is virtually pure fat, and those sensitive to fish often find they can take fish oils, which also contain no protein. The foods to which you are most likely to react are:

- wheat-based foods (see below for common foods usually made from or containing wheat)
- dairy foods (mainly cow's milk produce but you can also be sensitive to sheep or goat's milk products)
- gluten grains (see below)
- eggs – either egg white, yolk or both
- yeast
- soya
- chicken
- nuts – especially cashews, almonds, peanuts, Brazils
- kiwi fruit
- shellfish
- corn.

Foods Typically Made from or Containing Wheat

muesli	breadcrumbs
cous cous	some whiskies
bread	gravy
soya sauce	sausages
biscuits	many puddings
cakes	many sauces
pasta	batter
crackers	stock cubes
crispbreads	many breakfast cereals
pastries and pies	pizza
some beers	

Gluten-containing Grains

wheat	kamut
rye	triticale
oats	bulgar/cracked wheat
barley	semolina
spelt	

Wheat Intolerance

The most common culprits are, indisputably, wheat and dairy, with wheat intolerance being in my experience by far the most prevalent. I never fail to be astonished at how frequently wheat intolerance turns out to be the main offender. Removing the offender can often have an effect akin to waving a magic wand:

symptoms vanish. Sometimes these symptoms have plagued the individual in question for a lifetime. But there is a cause for everything, and once that cause is identified and removed, the healing process can begin.

Why is wheat such a frequent offender? First, the human body does not adjust readily to a new food and wheat is a relative newcomer to our diet in terms of human evolution (we started cultivating it around 10,000 years ago). Secondly, wheat has been engineered to such an extent that many people are simply not able to digest the gluten it contains. Gluten is a protein which makes bread doughy and heat-resistant and lends itself particularly well to breads, pastries, cakes and other modern-day staples. It is this gluten content which is incompatible with so many people. There are four main gluten-containing grains: wheat, rye, barley and oats. Each contains a different type of gluten and wheat gluten is a much more common offender than the gluten found in the other grains. Many people cannot tolerate wheat gluten, yet have no problem with other gluten-containing grains. However, an unfortunate few suffer from a severe form of gluten intolerance called coeliac disease.

In people with coeliac disease, gluten damages the gut lining, eroding the microscopic villi (finger-like protrusions) which line the intestinal wall and whose job it is to absorb nutrients from food. The result of villi erosion is malnutrition, weight loss, diarrhoea and weakness. Anyone with this condition needs to follow a strict gluten-free diet for life. Until only a few years ago the only way to diagnose coeliac disease was via a biopsy of the intestinal lining. Now, a simple blood test can reveal whether or not a patient has this condition.

Finally, when you consider how much of the stuff we eat, you begin to understand that wheat might cause a few problems. And we do tend to overdo the monotonous, wheat-rich modern diet: cereal or toast for breakfast, a sandwich for lunch and a quick bowl of pasta in the evening, day in, day out, constitute a recipe for reaction for the typical busy Briton for whom convenience and speed are paramount. Wheat is cheap and versatile so it is grown intensively, making its abundance a food manufacturer's dream.

You may suspect at this point that I am wheatist, but be assured I am not. I am not sensitive to wheat products myself, and can eat them with impunity (though prefer not to overdo it). I am, however, mildly dairy intolerant: most of the time it gives me no trouble, but if I go on a bit of a cheese-bender (I am totally addicted to cheese of any kind) I will develop eczema on my legs. The torturous itching is sufficient to make me renounce dairy for a few weeks, during which time the eczema clears up nicely, only to return the next time I fall off the cheese wagon.

Dairy Intolerance

Why are milk products so frequently indicted for health crimes? Well, designed by Nature exclusively for calves, cow's milk contains proteins which many people find hard to digest, and lactose (milk sugar) which causes problems for those who lack the enzyme (lactase) required to break it down. Lactase deficiency is not uncommon. Nor is it surprising when you consider that, once weaned off mother's milk, it is not entirely natural to switch to drinking the milk of another mammal, which is significantly different from human milk.

Lactose intolerance is fundamentally a metabolic abnormality, and does not involve the immune system. Typical symptoms of lactose intolerance include abdominal pain and diarrhoea, and excessive gas and bloating. In children it can cause middle ear infection (otitis media), asthma, eczema, rhinitis, hyperactivity and poor sleep. Your GP can arrange for you to have a lactose intolerance test if you suspect that you have this condition. On the plus side, you might be able to digest yoghurt and hard cheeses, such as parmesan, as these contain very little or no lactose.

On the odd occasion when a client tests positive to the dairy exclusion test (see below), his or her initial concern is for calcium intake. Nutritional orthodoxy has it that we should all eat plenty of dairy foods, because they are rich in calcium. That much is true, but doesn't explain why, when we consume so much dairy in the West, osteoporosis remains rife, compared to other countries where much less is consumed. The link between dairy foods and osteoporosis is a bone of contention in itself. To suggest avoiding dairy is no less than a nutritional heresy and we have been weaned onto the idea that, without the stuff, our bones would crumble like biscuits. The controversy continues to rage and remains unresolved. A scientific review of all the studies on dairy and bone health found that, although some studies found dairy to be beneficial, most found that it had no effect on bone health at all, and a few even found it to have a detrimental effect.[6] The good news for the dairy-intolerant is that there is plenty of calcium in other foods. You can get calcium from dark leafy greens such as watercress, kale, broccoli, spinach and rocket, and nuts and seeds – especially almonds and sesame seeds.

HOW TO IDENTIFY A FOOD INTOLERANCE

Some nutritional therapists – and many therapists of other disciplines, unfortunately – routinely advise all their clients to stop eating all wheat and dairy products, indefinitely. I totally disagree with this simplistic, blanket approach. First, it can make you feel wretched to have to avoid a food you really like, all the time. Wheat and dairy are two significant staples of the Western diet and you only need to avoid them completely if doing so noticeably improves your health. Secondly, you might be avoiding them for no good reason, if they have no discernibly negative effect on your health. That is not to say that I would recommend them in large amounts on a frequent basis to anyone. Refined wheat products – that is, the white stuff, such as pasta, white bread and pastries – have no real nutritional value. What's more, they can have a detrimental effect on blood-sugar levels (see Solution 2).

If you would like to identify any intolerances you may have, there are two systems you might want to consider: the exclusion test and the ELISA IgG blood test.

The Exclusion Test

This is considered the gold standard, and is indeed my preferred choice. The exclusion test works best with foods that are consumed frequently – that is, on most days. It is accurate and, what's more, costs nothing, other than a shot of willpower. There are a few variations on this theme, but I have found the system described below to work consistently well. Although I believe food intolerances to be fairly common, I believe *multiple* food intolerances to be fairly uncommon, so therefore do not see the need to routinely recommend expensive blood tests.

Here's how you do an exclusion test.

1. Keep a food diary for four to seven days. Write down everything you eat and drink throughout each day. Make sure the diary reflects your typical food intake – for accuracy's sake, it is best not to include days where you have deviated from the norm and eaten unusual foods. This

is a useful way of seeing just how much of any one food or drink you consume – you might find yourself shocked at just how much chocolate you eat, or how little water you drink throughout the day.

2. After the four to seven days, take a close look at your food diary. Are there certain foods you eat every day, such as bread or cheese? Perhaps you eat an egg sandwich every day at the office? In this case you might suspect both wheat and egg. Use coloured highlighter pens to mark the most likely offenders (listed on page 6) which make their way into your diet. Do you crave these foods? Decide which food is eaten the most frequently; this will be the food you will test first. I nearly always get my clients to start with wheat-based foods, because most people eat so much of the stuff.

3. Once you have decided which food you are going to eliminate (temporarily) from your diet first, do some preparation. Investigate alternatives (see page 14 for wheat alternatives) and stock up on foods which will be replacing your suspect. If you are avoiding dairy foods, you will need to avoid all milk, cheese, yoghurt and cream, and anything containing whey or casein (as these are milk proteins). This means reading food labels. You should also avoid produce made from sheep's or goat's milk – if you are sensitive to cow's milk there is the possibility that sheep and goat produce are OK, but for the purposes of this investigation it is best to exclude them. Please note that eggs do not fall into the 'dairy' category so you can continue to eat them during a dairy exclusion. Larger supermarkets and health

food stores stock soya, rice and oat milk, which make good alternatives to dairy milk. Sadly, there are no real alternatives to cheese. Soya 'cheese' is a travesty and best resisted, to avoid disappointment.

4. When you're ready, eliminate your chosen suspect for seven days. It is essential that you do this strictly, otherwise the test won't work. If you eat ready-meals, snacks or any other processed food, you absolutely must read Ingredients lists and make sure that they do not contain the food you are eliminating. Use the sample food diary on page 15 to monitor your results.

5. During the elimination period, keep a note of any symptoms and write these down in your diary. Do you find they are much improved, eliminated, or unchanged? How is your energy and general mood?

6. After seven days of avoiding the food under suspicion you can look forward to the test, which involves eating the food in question. Make yourself a nice big meal or snack containing that food. This is called the 'challenge'. So, for example, if you have avoided all wheat-based foods you could make some toast, a sandwich or a bowl of pasta. It does not matter if your dish contains other foods.

7. Eat and enjoy your meal or snack, but do not eat this challenge food again for at least another three days.

8. Wait and see what happens over the next two to three days. What happened after you reintroduced the food? Which, if any, of your symptoms returned, and how bad was the reaction? Write down this information in the diary.

Wheat-free Alternatives

100 per cent rye bread

100 per cent rye crispbread

porridge oats

oat cakes

barley

millet

corn and corn-based products, including corn pasta and polenta

potatoes and potato-based meals, such as potato and cucumber salad, baked potatoes with various fillings

rice and rice-based products, including rice cakes and rice noodles, rice pasta

quinoa

shop-bought or home-made muesli (made from oats, rice flakes, millet flakes, soya flakes, nuts, seeds, flaked almonds, desiccated coconut, dried fruit)

egg salad

beans and lentils (chickpeas in particular add tasty bulk to a meal)

mixed bean salad

buckwheat – inc. buckwheat pasta (despite the name, buckwheat is wheat-free).

tamari soya sauce (tastes the same as ordinary soya sauce but without the wheat)

NB Spelt, which has become popular of late, is still wheat, even though it contains less gluten than ordinary wheat. Therefore it should be avoided if excluding wheat.

Food Exclusion Diary

The foods below are suggestions – you can test any food you like	How did you feel when you avoided this food?	How did you feel and what symptoms did you experience when you reintroduced this food? (over the following 2–3 days)
All wheat-containing foods		
All dairy foods		
All gluten grains		
Chicken		
Soya produce		
Nuts (all or one particular suspect)		

Interpreting the Results

Clients often ask me how they will know they have an intolerance to the food they have tested, and I always tell them they will be left in no doubt. If you are sensitive to a food which you have avoided for a few days and then consume in copious amounts all in one sitting, your symptoms will manifest with a vengeance. So, for example, you may find that, several hours after eating the challenge food, your energy level plummets and you develop a bad headache. Alternatively you may find that, after a week of being IBS-free, your stomach bloats and you have pain and flatulence more debilitating than pre-test levels. Interestingly, the stronger your intolerance to a food, the greater your reaction will be after you reintroduce it into your diet. If you get a positive reaction which leaves you in no doubt that you and the food in question are incompatible, you should continue to avoid it.

Obviously, if nothing much changes when you are avoiding your prime suspect, and nothing much changes when you reintroduce it, you can assume that you don't have a sensitivity to that particular food. If this is the case there is no reason why you should continue to eliminate it from your diet, although I would not recommend heavy dependence on any one food for fear of developing an intolerance to it in the future. Furthermore, if you always eat the same food, you always get the same nutrients, which means you may not get the full range of nutrients your body requires.

Once you have established the results, you may wish to repeat the test, this time with another food you have placed under suspicion. You can challenge just about any food you like. I do not recommend testing more than one food at a time because, as well as drawing heavily on your willpower reserves, you will be left uncertain as to which food is the actual culprit. There is also the possibility that, after carrying out a couple of exclusion tests, you may decide that food intolerance isn't your particular nemesis, in which case you ought to consider investigating another dietary cause of your health issues. At least you will have eliminated one possibility, which brings you closer to your goal.

On the whole, avoiding one type of food is not such an onerous task. You just find palatable alternatives. Often when I suggest to a client that he or she may be sensitive to wheat and that an exclusion test is advisable, the first reaction is one of wild-eyed panic, as if I had just suggested a water fast wearing only sackcloth. Nearly always, even the most entrenched eating habits can be modified; clients frequently return with tales of newly discovered and much preferred provender, such as the alternatives to wheat-based products listed on page 14.

Frequently, people find that their symptoms improve, but do not vanish. I interpret this as meaning one of two things. Either you have further food sensitivities in addition to the one you've just identified, or there is more than one root cause of your health problems. If, for example, your symptoms improve but do not disappear when you are off wheat, you might want to consider the possibility that you are gluten sensitive, or dairy sensitive – just take a look at your food diary and see which foods you have highlighted. Once you have exhausted all possibilities as far as obvious food intolerance is concerned, you'll have to consider other possible causes, as outlined in the chapters that follow.

The Blood Test

This method of food intolerance testing costs a not inconsiderable sum of money but is fast, virtually painless and requires no willpower. Another great thing about this test is that you can take your own blood sample – a small finger prick suffices – and send it off for analysis yourself. This method works well for less ubiquitous foodstuffs than those listed above, but whose effects may be equally pernicious. I favour this approach when I believe multiple sensitivities are at play, and when the more obvious suspects have already been tested using the exclusion method, and eliminated from enquiries. Therefore I find I recommend the blood test quite rarely. As far as I am concerned, it comes a poor second to the exclusion test.

Known as the IgG ELISA (enzyme-linked immunosorbent assay) test, a sample of blood is tested for the presence of IgG antibodies to foods. Antibodies, as you may recall, are created by the body's immune system to fight what it perceives to be an enemy invader. So the presence of antibodies in the blood in readiness to deal with the enemy food is an indicator of food intolerance.

By avoiding offending items altogether (for at least four months) it is possible to grow out of an IgG sensitivity – the immune system simply 'forgets' to react to them and no longer identifies them as the enemy.

Case History

Caroline, a 45-year-old housewife, came to see me because she had been suffering from myriad symptoms that remained unresolved after years of futile investigations. Her main concern was her stomach pains – she regularly suffered from lower abdominal pain, accompanied by bloating and constipation. As well as digestive problems, she suffered from regular headaches and insomnia. Her food diary revealed that she typically ate toast or a wheat-based cereal for breakfast, a ham or tuna sandwich for lunch and meat, vegetables and potatoes for dinner – often with bread.

I asked Caroline to do a wheat exclusion test for seven days. We didn't meet until about six weeks later due to her various commitments, but when we did meet, she remarked on the changes she'd noticed straight away – her insomnia cleared up soon after starting the elimination so she stayed off wheat and she was now sleeping very well. Her abdominal pain and bloating had gone, her bowel movements were regular, on a daily basis, and her headaches had vanished. She also commented on her weight loss – 5 to 6 lb – with which she was 'absolutely delighted'. Weight loss is not unusual in wheat-sensitive people who start to avoid wheat – I encounter this all the time. Before you renounce all wheat, however, bear in mind that much of this loss is water, not fat.

Caroline felt much better off wheat – she commented that everything felt 'calmer'. She certainly wasn't going hungry: her typical diet now included yoghurt with puréed fruit for breakfast, avocado and prawn salad and soup for lunch, and chicken, potatoes and mixed vegetables for dinner.

FURTHER INVESTIGATIONS

See Solution 8: Healing a Leaky Gut if you have or believe you have multiple food sensitivities. Leaky gut (or intestinal permeability) is a condition which predisposes you to a multitude of possible food sensitivities, because damage to the gut lining allows undigested food particles to pass into the bloodstream and trigger an immune response.

Solution 2

Rebalancing Blood Sugar

An inability to maintain even blood-sugar levels throughout the day is, to my mind, one of the most common causes of those niggling health problems which beset most people who are supposedly healthy but in reality functioning below par. I say this with confidence: I find, almost invariably, that once action is taken to stabilize blood sugar levels, hitherto immutable symptoms just vanish.

Mention blood sugar and most people immediately think of diabetes. Diabetes is indeed the worst-case scenario when it comes to blood-sugar imbalance (BSI). It is a serious condition requiring medical intervention.

BSI, on the other hand, is not a medical condition in itself and although the path to diabetes is paved with BSI symptoms, most people with BSI do not, happily, go on to develop diabetes. But some do, and the number is increasing.

Whenever BSI emerges as the most likely culprit during a consultation, I know I am probably onto a winner because in most cases it is by far the easiest cause to address. Clients will frequently report that they experience relief from symptoms within a few days of implementing their new dietary programme.

COMMON SYMPTOMS

These are the signs and symptoms you are most likely to experience if BSI is the source of your troubles:

- regular and inexplicable fatigue

- apathy

- mood swings

- poor memory and/or concentration

- food cravings (especially for sweet foods)

- difficulty waking up in the morning

- depression

- anxiety

- irritability

- cold hands and/or feet

- headache

- weight gain around the middle.

A key question I always ask each client whenever I suspect BSI is: How do you feel if you have to go several hours, say four or five, without eating? Frequently, the client will state categorically that he or she simply could not endure prolonged periods without eating, for fear of inducing headaches, mental confusion, light-headedness, irritability or tremor.

Before I incriminate BSI as the most likely cause of a client's health problems, however, I closely study his or her food diary. Have a look yourself at the food diary below, presented to me by a client and typical of someone with BSI. Does it bear any resemblance to your own typical diet?

Client's Food Diary

Breakfast

toast and jam, or

cornflakes with milk, or

nothing

cup of coffee

Mid-morning

cup of tea

flapjack

Lunch

cheese and tomato baguette or

mixed leaf, avocado and tomato salad

packet of crisps

Mid-afternoon

cup of coffee

apple

chocolate bar

Dinner

pasta with vegetarian sauce and a green salad or

chicken, rice (white) and peas or

baked potato with a variety of fillings, either vegetarian or fish-based

slice of cake

cup of tea

Before we discuss how this unremarkable diet can create such mayhem, let us first examine the role of blood sugar in maintaining health, and the medical conditions associated with blood-sugar disorder.

ABOUT BLOOD SUGAR

People rightly associate sugar with energy. Sugar – or more precisely glucose – provides fuel. It's in your blood and much of it fuels your brain. Without glucose, cognitive function is impaired: you can't think straight.

This glucose comes from the carbohydrates that you eat, although it is also manufactured from protein in the diet. Carbohydrates include starchy foods such as potatoes, bread, pasta, rice and other grains, beans, lentils, fruits and vegetables. These carbohydrates are broken down by the digestive system into simple sugars which are then able to cross the gut lining and enter the bloodstream. Like most things, you need glucose in just the right amounts; too little or too much are both potentially perilous. Typically, you should have about a teaspoon's worth coursing through your entire system at any given time.

Raised glucose levels stimulate the production in the pancreas of a hormone called insulin. The more carbohydrate we eat, the more insulin is produced. Protein also stimulates insulin production, but to a much lesser degree. Insulin lowers glucose by delivering it to the muscles and organs to provide them with the energy they need to carry out their normal functions. Any excess glucose is stored in the form of glycogen in the liver, or in the muscles for future use. If these stores are already full, it will be accumulated as fat.

If your blood-sugar levels should fall, the hormone glucagon, also secreted by the pancreas, helps restore balance by drawing on your reserves of glycogen held in the muscles and liver. That, at least, is what happens in the ideal terrain. When blood-sugar regulation goes seriously awry, there are two main conditions you might develop: type 2 diabetes and insulin resistance.

Diabetes

There are two types of diabetes: type 1 and type 2. In type 1, the pancreas is unable to secrete insulin. Regular insulin injections are an essential part of treatment. About 5 to 15 per cent of all people with diabetes have type 1, the cause of which remains unknown.

Type 2 is different. It is much more common and is linked to diet and lifestyle, and occurs when the body is unable to make sufficient insulin, or to use the available circulating insulin. When blood sugar is consistently higher than it should be, there is intensified pressure on the pancreas to pump out insulin in ever greater amounts in order to meet demand. Consequently the pancreas can become exhausted and stop working properly. It isn't hard to figure out: if you have the equivalent of a teaspoon of sugar circulating in your bloodstream, and then you eat a bar of chocolate that has around 12 teaspoons of sugar, then wash that down with a can of cola that has around eight teaspoons, your pancreas will be fired into overdrive in order to produce enough insulin to deal with this sickly sweet onslaught. Imagine doing this to yourself every day, as many people do. For ever-increasing numbers of people, type 2 diabetes is the result. The pancreas becomes exhausted, no longer able to cope with the heavy demands placed upon it.

Incidence of type 2 diabetes is snowballing, and what is particularly concerning is the fact that it is now affecting children, which until a few years ago was virtually unheard of. What was once referred to as 'adult-onset' diabetes has widened its net to become more inclusive. Initially observed in the US in the 1990s, reports of the condition manifesting in children in Europe and elsewhere emerged about a decade later.[1] This is in part due to the fact that obesity is a significant risk factor in type 2 diabetes: in the UK nearly 14 per cent of children aged between two and ten are now classified as obese.

The two most common symptoms of diabetes are frequent urination and unabated thirst. Those with untreated diabetes may also experience blurred vision, fatigue and weight loss. Obviously if you suspect you may have diabetes you should stop reading this now and head off to your GP forthwith, and get yourself tested.

Insulin Resistance

Also known as Syndrome X, or the 'metabolic syndrome', insulin resistance is a blood-sugar disorder just a step away from diabetes. Like diabetes, incidence of this condition is escalating. It occurs when the body's cells no longer respond adequately to insulin, as a result of long-term peaks and troughs in blood-sugar levels. It's as if the body's cells have become immune to insulin, which has lost much of its potency. Essential as insulin is, like anything that is good, in excess it is not so good. As high levels remain in the blood, the pancreas pumps out even more of the hormone in a futile effort to lower blood sugar. High insulin levels inhibit the breakdown of fat stores in the body, thus preventing weight loss. If you're wondering whether you have this condition, one clue is that, if you have, you will typically store fat around your middle (central obesity). Obesity is a causative factor in insulin resistance, and at the same time insulin resistance increases the risk of developing obesity. That's because high circulating blood glucose levels prevent your body from using its supply of fat as energy.

If you have insulin resistance, it's not just a fat tum you have to concern yourself with. High levels of circulating insulin increase the risk of developing a number of diseases including type 2 diabetes and heart disease.[2] Insulin promotes the production of fatty acids in the liver, which increases the amount of fat and LDL ('bad') cholesterol circulating in the blood. Unfortunately there's more: excessive levels of circulating insulin are also linked to atherosclerosis (furred-up arteries),[3] high blood pressure,[4,5] stroke,[6] polycystic ovaries,[7] Alzheimer's[8] and cancer.[9]

DO YOU HAVE A BLOOD-SUGAR IMBALANCE?

You may not have diabetes or insulin resistance, but there is a good chance you have BSI if the symptoms listed on page 22 look more than a little familiar and the diet outlined on page 23 bears more than a passing resemblance to your own. This diet is high in sugar and refined carbohydrates, and low in protein – protein is key to maintaining even blood-sugar levels. Do you find it hard to go extended periods without eating, or find you crave sweet foods? If so, this may be further evidence that you are struggling to maintain even blood-sugar levels.

In order to establish whether or not your blood-sugar levels are on an even keel, I recommend you keep a food diary for at least three days, and make sure that these days are typical of your eating patterns. Once done, compare your eating habits with those described below, which are those most likely to induce BSI:

- skipped meals, especially breakfast

- carbohydrate-rich meals with little or no protein and/or fat

- high intake of refined carbohydrates

- frequent snacking on sugar-rich foods such as biscuits or chocolate bars

- added sugar in hot drinks or on breakfast cereals

- regular intake of soft drinks

- low fibre intake (fewer than five portions of fruit and vegetables daily).

HOW DOES IT ALL GO SO WRONG?

Diet is everything. Through diet you can either achieve healthy, balanced blood sugar or start an internal fuel crisis. Clients regularly tell me they eat sugary foods in order to get some energy. Sometimes their GP has told them to do this. These people have terrible energy levels, but because they equate sugar with energy, doggedly persist in consuming the very stuff which is creating their fatigue. Foods which contain added sugar (usually in the form of glucose or sucrose) are certain to cause a sudden rise in blood sugar, so in our example outlined on page 23, jam, cornflakes, flapjacks, chocolate bars and cake can all be incriminated. So too can the refined carbohydrates such as white bread, white rice and white pasta, all starchy foods which have been stripped of their fibre content, denatured and denuded of any goodness they once contained so that what is left is simple sugar. You may well enjoy the sugar rush, but, as you probably know, it is short-lived. As your raised blood-glucose levels crash from a height, so do you. And it is whilst you are down there in the sugar doldrums, feeling irritable, worn out and unable to think clearly, that you crave your next fix. You're stuck in a sugar loop.

WHAT TO DO ABOUT IT

Sugar is undeniably addictive. You are not born with a sweet tooth, but if you persevere long enough you can certainly develop one. On the plus side, your cravings can be overcome relatively quickly and blood sugar rebalanced fairly easily: you should notice improvements in symptoms within just a few days of making appropriate dietary changes. These changes are hardly torturous. You might take fright at the idea of weaning yourself off sugar, but I can honestly say that the vast majority of people I see do not actually find this to be as challenging as they originally anticipated. In my experience I have found that it takes most people less than a week to wean themselves off their addiction.

So, assuming you are now convinced that you need to balance your blood-sugar levels, your priority is to sort out your diet and ensure a steady supply of energy throughout the day.

Dietary Changes for Balanced Blood-sugar and Energy Levels

Do Not Skip Meals

And especially do not skip breakfast. Having said that, many people – myself included – do not feel like a feast first thing in the morning. That's fine: have a late breakfast instead, but don't leave the house without having eaten at least some fruit or a few unsalted nuts. You don't want to be one those people who passes out on the bus or tube on the way to work because his or her blood sugar is too low to maintain an upright position.

Eat Protein with Each Meal

Protein is essential for balancing blood sugar and reducing insulin resistance. It is especially important that there is a protein component to your breakfast, otherwise you may trigger blood-sugar problems which last all day. Proteins are also essential for the manufacture of neurotransmitters in the brain, so without a breakfast supply you may find that 'thinking straight' is much harder than usual.

Protein Foods

- fish

- meats

- eggs (go for organic – the fat content is better. See Solution 4 for more details on this)

- dairy – cheese, yoghurt

- nuts and/or seeds. The plain, unsalted variety. For nuts try cashews, Brazils, hazelnuts, almonds. Tasty seeds include pumpkin and sunflower

- beans and lentils. Fantastic foods with a low glycaemic index (see below). Normal tinned baked beans tend to be sugar-laden; try the sugar-free variety now commonly available. Also try chick peas, kidney, haricot, cannellini, butter, black, adzuki … Any bean is good, even tinned as long as sugar hasn't been added. Green or puy lentils make a versatile and delicious alternative to the usual round of potatoes, rice or pasta

- soya produce – e.g. tofu. Marinated tofu is rather tasty, if you find the plain stuff a tad bland.

Avoid Adding Sugar to Anything

If you can give up sugar in your tea or coffee, do so. Most people find it takes them two to three days to get used to going without, after which time they find the idea of sweetened hot drinks repulsive. Don't even think of using artificial sweeteners. They are horrible chemicals which your body can live without and which are suspected carcinogens (cancer-causing agents). Cakes, biscuits and chocolate are out, for the time being. If you are a sugar addict, I suggest you go cold turkey for about a month. By the end of that time you'll have lovely, even blood-sugar levels and will probably have found your cravings have long since left you. As a bonus, you should be able to have the occasional chocolate/biscuit/slice of cake without feeling as though your life depended on it.

Follow a Low-Glycaemic Index (GI) Eating Programme

More on this below. Now, there have been countless eating plans which have come and gone, and they have mostly fallen by the wayside once people have come to their senses and realized that they were at best ineffective and at worst dangerous. The GI way of eating is not one of them; it's one of the healthiest diets there is. It is usually, and quite rightly, associated with weight loss. It is an excellent way of shedding excess pounds. But that is not usually why I recommend it. It was originally devised for people with diabetes, because it can help stabilize blood sugar in those with type 2. It is also now known to help prevent heart disease, and stabilize mood. A low-GI diet has been found to reduced LDL ('bad') cholesterol and reduce blood pressure. It is just fantastic – indeed, the World Health Organization recommends it as a diet for everyone.[10]

Eat Lots of Antioxidant-rich Foods

Antioxidants are nutrients which counter the harmful effects of chemicals in the body, known as free-oxidizing radicals, which are created by pollution, smoking, drinking alcohol and eating fried foods. Antioxidants negate the effects of this oxidative stress which, although a normal side effect of burning oxygen in the body, is believed to be a major contributor to insulin resistance.

So to fight off these free radicals, eat lots of plant foods in the form of fruits and vegetables, especially those which have bright or deep colours (peppers, red onion, oranges, plums, carrots, etc.). It is the pigment in these colourful plants which is laden with antioxidants. Dark leafy greens are also antioxidant-rich, so make spinach, broccoli, greens and so on part of your regular diet.

Exercise!

It is well established that exercise – whether it be of the intense, short-burst or endurance variety – improves glucose tolerance and insulin action.[11] Regular, moderate exercise encourages more effective insulin function. You know it makes sense: exercise is essential for whole body health, as it stimulates all the body's systems. So aim to exercise most days for about an hour. What you do is entirely up to you and your preferences – the only imperative is that you do what you enjoy, because if it's an ordeal you are not likely to stay the course.

THE GLYCAEMIC INDEX AND THE GLYCAEMIC LOAD

The glycaemic index is a system which measures the speed at which the carbohydrate component of food enters the bloodstream and raises blood sugar, on a scale of 0 to 100.

Carbohydrates are categorized as having either a low, medium or high GI. A low GI is a score of 55 or less, a medium GI score is 56–69 and a high GI score is 70 or over. Therefore, you want to avoid high-GI foods as much as possible and aim to eat mainly low GI foods with some medium scorers.

The glycaemic load (GL) takes the GI a step further. It looks at the GI of the overall food, not just its carbohydrate content. It is thought to be a more accurate measurement than the GI. For example, consider watermelon. The sugar content of watermelon has a high GI content, but the whole fruit itself actually contains very little sugar – much of the fruit is water. So although it has a high GI (72) it has a low GL score (4).

You can calculate the GL of a food by multiplying the GI by the grams of carbohydrates per serving, divided by 100 – but frankly I don't recommend this. You don't want to become obsessed with this system, and therefore food, in the way that people become obsessed with counting calories, or weighing portions. It simply isn't healthy. Just remember this rule of thumb: all fruits and vegetables are good, and can and should be consumed in copious amounts. They have a low GL because they generally have a high-water, low-sugar content. This does not include juices, which are stripped of fibre and therefore have a much higher GL. For foods other than fruits and vegetables, just refer to the table below. Different GI tables may show a slight variation in scores; the rating depends on the cooking and processing methods used, so some variation is inevitable.

Perhaps one reason why the GI diet is so healthy is that it is not a million miles away from the hunter-gatherer way of eating. Our hunter-gatherer ancestors did not farm; we only started doing so around 10,000 years ago – a mere blink of the eye in terms of human evolution. Therefore grains such as wheat, corn and rice are newcomers to the human diet. Virtually all snack foods are made from these grains, or from potatoes – all of which have very high GI scores. The snack food industry relies heavily on our consumption of high-GI carbohydrates. They feed our addiction whilst we feed theirs. Refined carbohydrates are cheap and have been mass-produced ever since the Industrial Revolution. It's just not how the human animal was designed to eat. So get in touch with your inner hunter-gatherer and go for meat, fish, eggs, loads of fruits and vegetables, beans and lentils. If you eat bread, keep it to a minimum and only have wholemeal. Don't have toast on its own for breakfast – have it with a protein food such as eggs, or perhaps some peanut butter. See the Meal Ideas chapter for foods suitable for blood-sugar balancing.

Like most things, it's all about balance. Carbohydrates are important and should not be cut out of the diet, and you can never overdo the fruits and vegetables. People tend to forget that fruit and veg are carbohydrates too, and along with beans and lentils are rich in fibre. Fibre plays an important role in maintaining even blood sugar by holding onto the sugar content of a carbohydrate and releasing it slowly into the bloodstream. Think of the effect of refining a carbohydrate as a bit like destroying the natural environment by chopping down trees, thereby predisposing that environment to flooding. As outside, so inside. Note that cereal grains, even wholegrain cereals, tend to be on the high end of the GI index. Rice has an especially high GI, so be very cautious about including this in your diet if you are aiming to balance blood-sugar levels.

The Glycaemic Index of Foods

Please note that the GI is the same, whatever the quantity of a given food.

Low-glycaemic food	Rating
mushrooms	9
peanuts	13
green leafy vegetables	15
soya beans	18

Low-glycaemic food	Rating
fructose (fruit sugar)	23
cherries	24
grapefruit	25
pearl barley	25
kidney beans	29
butter beans	31
apricots	31
strawberries	32
chickpeas	33
yoghurt	33
pears	36
wholemeal (brown) pasta (spaghetti)	37
apples	38
haricot beans	38
fish fingers	38
plums	39
apple juice	41
porridge made with water	42
peaches	42
oranges	44
grapes	46
peas	48
baked beans	48

Low-glycaemic food	Rating
carrots (boiled)	49
kiwi fruit	52

Medium-glycaemic food	Rating
banana	55
muesli	56
pitta bread	57
white spaghetti	58
basmati rice	58
sweetcorn	59
pizza	60
ice cream	61
cous cous	65
melon	65
sucrose (table sugar)	65
shredded wheat	67
croissant	67
Mars bar	68
Ryvita	69
wholemeal bread	69
Weetabix	69

High-glycaemic food	Rating
white bread	70
boiled potatoes	70
bagel	72
baked potato	72
Cheerios	74
corn chips	74
chips	75
doughnut	76
brown rice	76
water biscuits	78
puffed wheat	80
Rice Crispies	82
rice cakes	82
instant mashed potatoes	83
pretzels	83
Cornflakes	84
popcorn	85
white rice	90
baguette	95
Lucozade	95
glucose	100

Case History

I have managed more cases of BSI than anything else, so the number of case histories I could describe is overwhelming. I have settled on Valerie, as she was so typical of my clients with BSI. I must have seen hundreds just like her and, just like Valerie, they were stunned at how quickly their symptoms cleared up, just by following a regimen designed to balance blood sugar.

Valerie was only 22 but came with a symptom list as long as her arm. She had trouble sleeping, felt tired all the time ('permanently lethargic' was how she described herself), had a cluster of premenstrual symptoms including cravings and bloating, was often irritable for no good reason and had poor concentration. Other than that, she was technically disease-free. She was a few pounds overweight and regularly craved sweet foods. This was what she typically ate and drank:

- *Breakfast:* white toast and honey, followed by a cup of tea
- *Lunch:* prawn salad, followed by a slice of lemon cake
- *Dinner:* mushroom burger with stir-fried vegetables. Chocolate bar. Half a bottle of wine.

Not the worst diet in the world, but certainly not the best. Note that there is no protein with breakfast, nor with the evening meal. What's more, there is no fruit, which makes it hard to achieve the recommended five-a-day portions of fruit and vegetables (and therefore antioxidants). There is plenty of sugar, though: cakes and chocolate ensure plenty of peaks and troughs, morning noon and night. Valerie didn't drink nearly enough water, which is bad enough in itself but worse still with a high-sugar diet, as sugar requires considerable amounts of water to be metabolized.

Valerie was also typical in that I was confident she could expect results almost immediately if she followed basic dietary guidelines. I explained the GI diet and advised at least six portions of fruit and vegetables daily. Pine nuts, sunflower and pumpkin seeds were to be eaten as snacks, and protein was to be eaten at each meal. Valerie was not vegetarian, so eating meat, fish, eggs and occasional dairy foods was not a problem. Out went the sugary snacks and chocolate. Alcohol was reduced to one glass of wine per day, with the evening meal.

One month later Valerie was back, but this was a new, improved Valerie. Her energy was now 'really good', her PMS that month had almost vanished, her sleep was almost normal and her irritability and other nervous symptoms had cleared up. Without actually aiming to do so, she had lost 3 lb in weight. She felt great and, like everyone else with similar symptoms, she was amazed at the speed of the results. I asked her what she personally felt had contributed the most to her quantum leap of health, and she was quite certain about this:
— Eating more protein and ditching the sugar. —

FURTHER INVESTIGATIONS

See Solution 3: Overcoming Adrenal Fatigue. If you are well and truly stressed, and have been for quite a while, you may need to consider adrenal fatigue as a causative factor. Adrenal fatigue is very much linked to BSI, as overproduction of adrenal hormones can increase insulin resistance.

Solution 3

Overcoming Adrenal Fatigue

If ever there was a word which resonates on a global level and which applies to all our lives, virtually on a daily basis, it has to be *stress*. Every day we face the stress of getting up, going out, confronting others, getting from A to B, doing difficult or tedious jobs, shopping, making our way home, settling domestic disputes, cooking and then attempting to get some sleep.

It's a tough old world and that's exactly how it's going to stay for the foreseeable future. Even those of us lucky enough not to live in a war zone sometimes feel as if we do. You know there are people far worse off than yourself, but that doesn't mitigate your own personal hardships and battles.

Chronic stress is emerging as a consequence of an unsustainable way of life in Britain today. The British work the longest hours in the EU, but all this productivity feeds a false economy when you consider that, according to the Health and Safety Executive, around half a million people in the UK are so stressed out by work alone that they believe it is making them ill.[1] It is certainly keeping them awake. A study conducted by the

Future Foundation for the British Association for Counselling and Psychotherapy found that almost a third of the population regularly suffers from lack of sleep, with anxiety as the most cited reason.[2] Put that stressed-out, sleepless individual behind the wheel and you see why Britain holds the world title for road rage.[3]

It may be unwelcome but stress is the norm, and indeed can have a positive effect on human creativity and productivity. Who would really want to live a life devoid of challenges? The problem is that people are just not coping with life's slings and arrows, and are therefore suffering the consequences. You may not think that diet plays much of a role in the body's coping mechanisms, but think again. Your body is hard-wired to deal with stressful situations, given the right nutritional terrain. What you eat can have a profound effect on how your body deals with mental stressors, as we shall see.

ANATOMY OF STRESS

There is stress, and then there is stress. It was the world authority on the subject and author of *The Stress of Life* (1956), Hans Selye, who first identified a common response to stress which he called the 'General Adaptation Syndrome'. According to Selye, humans and animals respond in three stages when under extreme stress. These are:

1. the alarm reaction, when your body goes on full alert. Stress is detected and the body reacts by producing adrenaline.

2. adaptation, or resistance. You adapt to and learn to cope with the stressor.

3. exhaustion. You are no longer able to deal with the stress and resistance has greatly declined.

The body's response to stress is activated by what is called the hypothalamic-pituitary-adrenal (HPA) axis. The hypothalamus is a gland in the brain which stimulates and controls the pituitary gland in response to the changes it detects, and in turn the pituitary stimulates production of hormones by the adrenal glands. You are equipped with two adrenal glands, one on top of each kidney, and these produce hormones in response to stressful situations or thoughts.

STAGE ONE – THE BEGINNING

During stage one, the hormones adrenaline and noradrenaline are released as a sort of 'knee-jerk' reaction to a given situation. This prepares you for 'fight or flight' and is short-term only. Stored glycogen is converted to glucose, so blood sugar rises and the flow of fatty acids into the bloodstream also increases, to give you more energy to fight or flee. The heart pumps faster to get more oxygen and nutrients to muscles, and energy is routed away from non-essential functions, such as digestion. Breathing rate increases and the respiratory passageways widen to accommodate more air, and therefore more oxygen. Even blood-clotting agents are mobilized, in case you are wounded. This alarm reaction is nothing less than a spectacular feat of biochemical engineering, and it is a pity that you are unable to appreciate its sublimity when in operation. We may be living in the 21st century as far as our external environment is concerned, but we still inhabit Stone Age bodies, with the same internal structures as our Neolithic forebears. Our nervous and hormonal systems do not distinguish between stress of the wild-beast-intent-on-devouring-us type, or the vile-boss-making-unreasonable-demands type. The response is always the same.

STAGE TWO – STRESS SETTLES IN

The adrenaline response works in the short term, but in the long term – stage two – the body uses other hormones to deal with prolonged, unrelenting stress, long after the effects of the alarm stage have dissipated. During the second, or adaptation stage, activation of the HPA axis stimulates production of the hormone cortisol, and excessive cortisol production is a key feature of stage two of the stress response. Normally, this hormone is produced cyclically in what is termed the *circadian rhythm*: levels start to rise between 3 a.m. and 6 a.m. and gradually decrease throughout the day, so that by night-time they are at their lowest.

Like most essential things, cortisol is required in just the right amounts: too little, or too much, can disturb the homeostasis of the body. Why is cortisol so important? You need this hormone because it:

- stimulates the conversion of protein and fat to glucose for energy, thus increasing blood-sugar levels
- stimulates the release of fatty acids from fat cells to be used as fuel for energy
- stimulates cellular repair
- increases mental and physical energy
- has a powerful anti-inflammatory effect
- improves mood
- reduces the allergic response
- controls the immune system – it prevents overreaction of white blood cells which could lead to autoimmune disease (where the body attacks its own cells and organs)
- maintains blood pressure by preventing sodium loss.

During stage two the body produces cortisol in excess and, over a prolonged period, this surfeit can be detrimental to health. So too can excessive aldosterone, another adrenal hormone produced at this stage. Aldosterone raises blood pressure by retaining sodium in cells, which is why high blood pressure is often symptomatic of prolonged stress.

The effects of elevated cortisol include raised blood-sugar levels and all the problems this can cause (see Solution 2) and weakened immunity – virtually all components of the immune response are inhibited by cortisol.[4] This effect leaves you susceptible to colds, flu and other immune-related disorders. Elevated cortisol suppresses the secretion of growth hormone – important because it carries out repair work when you are asleep. Headaches, sleep disorders and heart disease can also result from excessive cortisol production, brought about by chronic activation of the HPA axis. Protein breakdown is increased, and this can lead to muscle wasting and osteoporosis. Cortisol is made from the female hormone progesterone so, not surprisingly, adrenal fatigue can disturb the menstrual cycle in women because prolonged stress can result in progesterone supplies being diverted to create cortisol.

And Another Thing ...

Among the principal misdemeanours of unrestrained cortisol is, as we have seen, its ability to create hormonal havoc. This is particularly true when it comes to another important adrenal steroid hormone, dehydroepiandrosterone, or DHEA. DHEA is the most abundant steroid found in the blood and is a precursor to other hormones including testosterone and oestrogen. It is produced abundantly until around the age of 20, when levels start to decline. It is effectively the hormone that keeps you young and slim. It's bad enough that secretion falls naturally as we age, without it being diminished even further by periods of unrelenting stress. Excessive cortisol diminishes the body's level of DHEA. DHEA is essential because it:

- stimulates the immune system and counters the effects of excessive cortisol

- lowers LDL ('bad') cholesterol

- can help prevent osteoporosis by stimulating bone deposition

- can help slow down the ageing process

- stimulates metabolism

- reduces the symptoms of premenstrual syndrome

- stimulates the burning of fat for fuel

- increases vitality

- boosts sexual function

- regulates mood.

STAGE THREE: CRASH, BURN, CRY

Although the resistance stage can last as long as several years, the body's capacity for adaptation has its limits, and if there is no let-up in the burden of mental trauma the exhaustion stage (also known as the adrenal maladaptation stage) is an inexorable fate. It is at this point that disproportionate cortisol output, which the adrenals can no longer sustain, starts to decline, falling to below normal levels. Mental and physical exhaustion ensue. This is not the same as Addison's disease, which is a rare, chronic and life-threatening condition which may involve structural damage to the adrenal gland and requires the patient to take corticosteroid medication for life. Most cases of Addison's are the result of tuberculosis infection or autoimmune disease, where the body attacks its own organs, leading to adrenal failure.

Chronic fatigue syndrome (CFS) and fibromyalgia (a condition characterized by musculoskeletal pain and fatigue), weakness and dizziness are all linked to cortisol insufficiency. Indeed, HPA axis dysfunction has been found to be present in the majority of patients with both CFS and fibromyalgia.[5] Giving low doses of cortisol has been shown to treat both conditions effectively.[6] Even so, adrenal exhaustion is still not widely recognized as a medical condition, despite increasing and compelling evidence that the adrenal glands can become underactive as a result of stress.[7] People suffering from post-traumatic stress disorder (PTSD) have been found to under-secrete cortisol, as have 'healthy' individuals living under conditions of chronic stress.[8]

DO YOU HAVE ADRENAL FATIGUE?

The person best qualified to identify stress as a factor in your levels of health and wellbeing is you. That is why, whenever I suspect that adrenal fatigue (sometimes referred to as adrenal stress) may be aggravating a client's symptoms, I ask: 'Are you very stressed out? And if so, has the stress in your life been going on for a long time?' If the client answers an unequivocal 'Yes,' I follow up with: 'Do you think stress is affecting your health, energy levels and sense of wellbeing?'

It is not uncommon, at this point, for my client to embark on a narrative of events, often starting in childhood. These stories are variously fascinating, heart-breaking, depressing and shocking, but they are always unique and always serve as a reminder to me of the human ability to withstand enormous challenges and stresses. But stress does eventually take its toll on mind and body, to varying degrees.

The reason why some people are able to deal with punishing stress levels for so long, whilst others succumb early to the detrimental effects of endless pressure, may lie in how well their adrenals are functioning.

As we have seen, adrenal fatigue is progressive. Stage one is normal – a fascinating display of the body's autonomic defence system which swings into action without your having to do anything of your own volition. Stages two and three are much more of a concern. If you are at stage two, your symptoms are likely to include:

- frequent headaches
- insomnia (because cortisol is high at night, when it should be low)
- menstrual irregularities
- frequent colds and infections
- signs of premature ageing.

If you are at stage three, your symptoms are likely to include:

- chronic fatigue
- painful muscles
- apathy
- weakness

- depression

- dizziness (especially on rising suddenly, because of low blood pressure).

At any stage of adrenal fatigue you are likely to be using stimulants such as caffeine and alcohol to prop yourself up. You are also likely to have abnormal blood-sugar levels and find yourself lurching from one cold or infection to another. You may find it difficult to get up in the morning and struggle with memory and concentration. Stressful situations become more difficult to handle and you find yourself becoming increasingly irascible. Despite this, you might be driving yourself forward, eating poorly and never taking the time to relax. I know this doesn't help right now, but you should be aware that you are also at increased risk of developing osteoporosis and heart disease later on, should the situation remain unresolved.

If, by now, you suspect that suboptimal adrenal function may be behind your symptoms, you will hopefully be inspired by the knowledge that you *can* do something about it. You can start by following the advice below on how to stabilize adrenal function through diet and lifestyle changes. You may also wish to take a salivary hormonal test known as an adrenal stress index, or ASI, which examines cortisol and DHEA levels throughout the day and identifies any excesses or deficiencies. I have always made good use of the ASI test, because it tells me not only if adrenal fatigue is a factor, but at what stage of adrenal stress my client has arrived. This test is very simple and can be performed at home – the laboratory posts a kit to you and you follow the instructions provided, which entail collecting four saliva samples at four different times of the day: 7–8 a.m., midday, 4–5 p.m. and 11 p.m.–midnight. You then send off your four vials and wait for the results to be posted to you. See the Resources chapter for details of a laboratory which carries out this test.

STABILIZING ADRENAL OUTPUT

Before embarking on a new dietary regime, you need to think seriously about the stress in your life and what you can do to minimize it. There is no one unique solution; the best approach embraces stress-management, relaxation techniques and, of course, dietary changes. Stress is one area where a truly holistic approach is imperative if you are to get effective results.

Stress Management

There are stress-management techniques you can adopt yourself, and techniques which require the help of others. Exercise is a good starting point because this is something you can initiate on your own. Exercise is important because it helps normalize levels of stress hormones in the blood, and improves circulation. It also stimulates the release of endorphins – 'happy hormones' – which can elicit a sense of wellbeing and positivity. Aerobic exercise stimulates the production of cortisol, so ideally should be carried out in the morning only, if cortisol is low. It is especially important that you do not engage in aerobic exercise in the evening, as normally cortisol levels should be falling at this time, in preparation for sleep. If you do not know if your cortisol is high or low, opt for gentle exercise only: daily walking, yoga, stretching or swimming. Whatever you do, it has to be something you enjoy.

Relaxation

In addition to exercise there are other effective tools you can utilize to manage stress levels. Your method of choice is a matter of what you feel drawn towards. Possibilities include meditation, positive imagery and deep-breathing techniques. You might prefer a regular massage, aromatherapy or reflexology. If you feel you need a talking therapy, you might want to consider some professional help from a stress counsellor.

Dietary Manipulation

The dietary regime designed to help stabilize the adrenals is essentially the same, whatever stage of adrenal stress you have succumbed to. Therefore you can follow the advice below regardless of whether or not you have taken the ASI test. Dietary management of adrenal stress is fairly straightforward and manageable and you should not find it too difficult to follow.

Your priority is stabilizing blood sugar. Achieving this takes the pressure off the adrenals and helps them normalize hormonal output. Fluctuations in blood sugar can stimulate cortisol output and are a stress on the body, but if you are not producing enough cortisol you are more likely to experience low blood sugar.

Full details of dietary management of blood sugar are given in the Solution 2 chapter. The most important dietary essential is the removal of all sugar and refined carbohydrates from the diet, and the inclusion of fat and protein with every meal. This will ensure that you are eating a low-glycaemic index diet. Examples of good dietary protein are also given in the Solution 2 chapter.

If there's one other dietary component you must have in your quest to normalize adrenal output, it's the fatty acids commonly known as omega-3 fatty acids, of the type found in oily fish. You can read all about the role of fatty acids in the Solution 4 chapter, but for now all you need to know is that these fats help stabilize HPA axis activity. Low levels of these fatty acids are associated with HPA axis overactivity,[9] and supplemental omega-3 has been found to inhibit adrenal activation triggered by mental stress.[10] The best omega-3 fish sources are sardines, salmon, herring, trout, mackerel, anchovies and tuna (fresh, not tinned). If you do not take fish oil supplements, I suggest you eat oily fish at least twice a week.

There are certain nutrients which are highly concentrated in the adrenals and which are essential for healthy adrenal function. In particular, the adrenals need vitamin C, B complex (especially B_5) and the mineral magnesium.

Some Important Adrenal Nutrients, Their Sources and Roles

Vitamin C	All fruits and vegetables, especially kiwi, strawberries, blueberries, dark leafy greens	Needed to make cortisol and, indeed, all adrenal steroid hormones. The more stressed you are, the more rapidly you use up circulating vitamin C, which is normally found in highly concentrated levels in the adrenals. Vitamin C is also crucial to the immune system – which is always compromised in adrenal stress.
Vitamin B_5	Most foods, especially all meats, tomatoes, eggs, mushrooms, milk	This is another vitamin also highly concentrated in the adrenal glands. It is needed to convert glucose into energy and synthesize adrenal hormones. Having said that, all the B vitamins are required for healthy adrenal function and, fortunately for us, they are often found together in food, especially meat.

Magnesium	Dark leafy greens, nuts and seeds	This is probably the most important mineral for adrenal health. It is known as the anti-stress mineral because of its calming effects. It is a natural muscle relaxant and helps promote sleep. It also helps provide the adrenals with the energy they need to function adequately.

It is one thing to know which nutrients are helpful in assisting the adrenals, but quite another to translate that knowledge into practice. See the Meal Ideas chapter for some excellent suggestions. Hopefully you can see what's most important: protein in the form of meat, fish, dairy or eggs with each meal, with lots of fruits and vegetables. I have not included potatoes as they have a high glycaemic index which means they quickly elevate blood-sugar levels. Some wholegrains can be incorporated into this dietary regime, but I tend to restrict these to no more than one portion a day. I prefer to include beans and lentils rather than grains as they are more nutritious, higher in protein and have a lower glycaemic index. All beans are good, but be wary of conventional tinned baked beans as these tend to be high in added sugar. Sugar-free varieties are available. To cook dried beans requires considerable commitment: they have to be soaked overnight and then boiled for several hours. This does have its advantages: dried beans are relatively cheap and you can make bean dishes in large quantities and then freeze them. However, most people, I find, would rather just open a tin. That's fine, from a nutritional perspective, but just make sure that your beans of choice are sugar-free. Personal favourites include chickpeas, black-eyed beans, haricot, cannellini, adzuki, kidney and butter beans. Lentils also make a good basis for a meal: green and brown lentils lend themselves particularly well to vegetable stir-fries with, say, chicken, beef or fish. Red or green lentils can be used to make dhal. You can also grate some cheddar cheese over cooked lentils for an excellent pro-adrenal meal.

Vegetarians and Vegans

Balancing blood sugar and normalizing adrenal output can be a bit tricky if you do not eat meat, fish or any other animal product. This is because animal foods are complete proteins which usually also contain fat. Both protein and fat delay and control the release of sugars into the bloodstream. Vegetarians may have to rely more on dairy products and eggs, and vegans more on soya produce, beans and lentils, nuts and seeds. See page 30 for a list of good protein foods, from both animal and plant sources.

If you do not eat fish, or take fish oil supplements, getting the omega-3 fatty acids you need is also that much more challenging. Certain nuts and seeds, especially flaxseed (also known as linseed) and pumpkin seeds are rich in omega-3 fats, but these are different to the omega-3 fats found in fish. That is because the omega-3 fats in nuts and seeds have to be converted by the body into the fatty acids known as EPA and DHA, in order to be of any use, and the body does not do this efficiently – in fact very little of the oil in nuts and seeds is converted to EPA or DHA. The advantage of fish oil is that it is a ready-made, plentiful source of both these fatty acids, so no conversion is necessary.

Dietary Supplements

If you have decided to go ahead with a saliva test, I would urge that you do so via a nutritional therapist, or that you consult a therapist once you have received the results. When it comes to taking supplements for adrenal stress, this is best done with professional guidance. Having said that, some supplements help balance adrenal output whether you have stage two or three adrenal fatigue. Other supplements can raise cortisol and others depress it, in which case it is obviously crucial that the right supplements are taken. Registered nutritional therapists are to be found on the website of the British Association for Applied Nutrition and Nutritional Therapy, details of which are found in the Resources chapter.

The table below outlines a good basic support programme which I tend to use whatever level of adrenal stress I am attempting to address. In addition to these, many people find the herbal remedies Siberian ginseng, rhodiola and ginger root to be very effective. These are considered to be 'adaptogens' in that they help the adrenals regulate normal hormonal output.

Basic Supplement Programme for Adrenal Support

Supplement	Dosage	Frequency
Vitamin C	500mg	twice daily with food
B Complex	containing 50mg of B_5	1 daily, with breakfast
Magnesium	containing 200mg elemental magnesium	1 daily, with dinner
Fish oil	1,000mg	twice daily with food

How long will all this take? Most nutritional therapists will advise that you can expect to spend a minimum of two months normalizing adrenal function. You should, however, start to be aware of improvements in symptoms within a month.

Case History

Julie was an especially interesting case. At the age of 45 she came to see me with not only a long list of symptoms which suggested adrenal fatigue but lots of other problems, too, including poor digestion and painful, heavy periods. The symptoms she described which made me immediately suspect adrenal stress were total fatigue, poor sleep, depression and anxiety, joint pain, poor memory and concentration and regular headaches. I asked Julie if she felt she was stressed, and her answer was an unequivocal Yes. Then I asked her how long she had been under excessive stress – and the answer was 25 years! It wasn't difficult to conclude that adrenal stress might be contributing to her symptoms.

On the digestion side, Julie regularly experienced bloating, diarrhoea (alternating with constipation), bad breath and flatulence. She also suffered from hay fever and asthma. It seemed I had my job cut out.

A glance at her food diary revealed that it was heavily loaded with carbohydrates and was low on protein. It was quite normal for her to eat nothing but cereals and other carbohydrates throughout the day, without consuming any protein until the evening. Fortunately I was able to persuade her to take the ASI test. Whilst we waited for the test results, I got her to make significant changes to her diet, which were all about balancing blood-sugar levels: three meals a day with protein at each meal, lots of oily fish and dark leafy greens and snacking on nuts and seeds. I did suspect that she might have a wheat intolerance as she ate the stuff morning, noon and night and had a lot of digestive symptoms. However, as she already had a lot of dietary changes to make in order to deal with the adrenal fatigue, I only asked her to reduce her wheat intake to once a day (see the Solution 1 chapter for more information on food intolerances).

Four weeks later, Julie returned for her follow-up consultation. Just by making the dietary changes suggested, her headaches had cleared up, which she described as 'very unusual'. Her digestive symptoms had all improved, though they had not gone away completely. Low energy and insomnia and other adrenal stress symptoms remained unchanged.

By the time of this second appointment, Julie's test results had arrived. They showed that she was, as I suspected, at the exhaustion stage. Both cortisol and DHEA levels were depressed throughout the day. No wonder she felt so awful. Diet alone wasn't going to be enough: in this case I was in no doubt that Julie required some quality supplements to help bring up her adrenal output and restore homeostasis. I recommended a high-strength multivitamin and -mineral, vitamin C, fish oil, magnesium and Siberian ginseng.

I also persuaded Julie at this point to do the wheat exclusion test (see page 11) to deal with her digestive symptoms.

Six weeks later, Julie returned. Her health had been transformed: she was sleeping well, cravings for sweet food had vanished, she had had no headaches and her energy was much better. On the digestion side, her bowels were regular, she had no diarrhoea, bloating or flatulence. She had also unexpectedly lost 5-6 lb in weight – and said she was 'absolutely delighted'. The wheat exclusion test had been positive, and as a result she had begun avoiding all wheat products. It was clear to me that the source of her health problems had been both wheat intolerance and adrenal fatigue.

OTHER THERAPIES

- Reflexology is an excellent therapy in that it aids relaxation. Other relaxing therapies such as massage are to be highly recommended. I also favour acupuncture as a means of stimulating low functioning glands and organs. See Resources.

Solution 4

Redressing Fatty Acid Deficiency

If you go to any supermarket and peruse the 'healthy options' section for any product, you will find that the 'healthy' boast is usually predicated on the product's low-fat, or even no-fat, credentials. Fat is the *bête noire* of the health enthusiast. Food manufacturers, keen to demonstrate their corporate concern for public health, have gone to great lengths to instil into the consumer psyche the belief that fat is heinous. *Only 1 per cent fat!* proclaims the packaging of something bland and bereft of nutritional value as well as fat. Despite assurances that these fatless foods are in fact 'delicious', our tastebuds suggest otherwise. Even so, we are prepared to sacrifice flavour in exchange for alleged health benefits. Time was when we judged a food by its smell, texture and appearance of freshness, rather than its fat content per gram.

No wonder, then, that fat deficiency figures on my list of major causes of common symptoms.

FAT IS GOOD

Fat may have a bad reputation, but its infamy is, on the whole, unjustified. It is one of the three important food groups (the other two being protein and carbohydrate), it is an essential component of your diet and avoiding it will damage your health and eventually lead to serious complications.

Of course too much fat is not good for anyone, and people can and frequently do eat too much of it; the same can be said for protein and carbohydrate. Fat is a complex issue: there are different types, with different functions. As we all know, fat is also totally delicious, and without it many dishes would not only leave us feeling hungry but also deprived of a pleasurable eating experience.

DIETARY FAT

The main type of dietary fat is in the form of *triglycerides*. A triglyceride is a combination of three fatty acids attached to a unit of glycerol (which is half of a sugar molecule) and can be either solid (fat) or liquid (oil). A fatty acid is made up of a straight chain of carbon atoms.

There are three main types of dietary fatty acid: saturated, hydrogenated, and unsaturated. They are classified according to how many hydrogen atoms are attached to the fat molecule. Foods tend to contain a variety of different fatty acids, but one type tends to dominate in each food.

Saturated Fatty Acids

These fat molecules are called 'saturated' because all of the carbon atoms are saturated with hydrogen atoms. Being saturated with hydrogen makes them solid, or fairly solid, at room temperature (for example, butter). They are mostly found in animal products, but some are found in plant sources, such as coconut. They are natural substances which the body recognizes and can process. Sources include meat and meat products, especially red meat, cheese and other dairy products such as cream and butter, lard, coconut oil, coconut cream and palm oil. Although often vilified, saturated fatty acids are useful to the body, especially the nervous system. They are an important component of grey matter and nervous tissue. Myelin, the insulating outer sheath which coats the nerve, is made firm by saturated fats. Although readily available from our diet, the body can also synthesize saturated fat if required.

Hydrogenated and Trans Fatty Acids

If any component of the modern diet genuinely deserves to be decried, castigated and stripped of rank before being unceremoniously booed offstage, it is hydrogenated fat. Hydrogenation is the process by which the double bonds on polyunsaturated fatty acids (see below) are *artificially* saturated with hydrogen, to make them solid. Hydrogenation significantly alters the shape of the fat molecule, straightening out its natural kink, thereby changing it from what is called a *cis* formation to a *trans* formation, a process which creates *trans fatty acids*.

In this regard, hydrogenated fats are the evil twin of saturated fats. Saturated fat has for too long unjustly taken the flak for the nefarious workings of its synthetic sibling. This fudging has meant that nutritionists have been distracted from the food industry's practice of merrily but quietly creating trans fatty acids and adding them to food products. These fatty acids have no nutritional value for the human body, which is designed to deal with cis formations, not trans formations.

The processed food industry is always keen to point out that meat and dairy products also contain trans fats. That much is true, but they contain very little, and the trans fats they do contain have different chemical structures than their industrially produced counterparts and are not alien to the human body.

It is not surprising, therefore, that the process of artificial hydrogenation has serious implications for human health. Trans fatty acids are perhaps most notorious for their link with heart disease. They increase blood platelet aggregation which can cause clotting.[1] They are associated with a higher risk for heart disease compared to saturated fats.[2] They are known to increase blood levels of LDL cholesterol (often referred to as 'bad' cholesterol) and decrease levels of HDL ('good') cholesterol. Trans fats are hypothesized to be carcinogenic, and although there is, to date, no conclusive evidence, studies suggest an association with colon cancer[3,4] and breast cancer.[5] In pregnant women, trans fats are able to cross the placenta and decrease birth weight.[6]

Another heinous hydrogenation crime to add to the above is the way that trans fatty acids interfere with the metabolism of both omega-3 and omega-6 fatty acids, making them less available to the body.[7] These are the essential fatty acids your body needs. You will see why it is so crucial to obtain these fatty acids from diet, and why it is therefore so important that you give trans fats a wide berth.

If hydrogenation and the subsequent creation of trans fats is so clearly detrimental, why do it in the first place? For profit and convenience, of course. Hydrogenation makes oil more useful for food processing because trans fatty acids solidify at room temperature and prolong shelf life and enhance flavour. They are most likely to be found in foodstuffs such as biscuits, cakes, ready-meals, pastry and some margarines. They have also been used, rather shamelessly, in some vegetarian foodstuffs purporting to be healthy. Fortunately that is now a less common occurrence, thanks to the bad publicity that hydrogenation has attracted over the last few years.

UK law at the moment states that trans fats do not have to be included in the nutritional information provided on a food label, and they do not need to be listed in the ingredients. However, hydrogenated vegetable oil must be declared in the ingredients list – so if you see 'hydrogenated' or 'partially hydrogenated' on the label, think trans fat. The good news is that Marks & Spencer, Waitrose, Sainsbury's, Tesco and ASDA all claim to have removed hydrogenated fats from all their own-brand products. To be fair to food manufacturers, many have now stopped using hydrogenated fats in their products, but I regularly peruse labels in supermarkets and still occasionally come across this egregious ingredient.

Unsaturated Fatty Acids

These are called 'unsaturated' because at least one carbon atom in the chain is not saturated with hydrogen. Instead, there is a double bond between carbon atoms. An unsaturated fatty acid may be either *monounsaturated* (which means there is one double bond in the fatty acid chain) or *polyunsaturated* (meaning there are two or more double bonds in the fatty acid chain).

Monounsaturated Fatty Acids

These are liquid at room temperature, but still quite dense; they start to solidify if refrigerated (think what olive oil looks like on a cold day). Monounsaturates (sometime referred to as omega-9 fats) are believed to be heart-friendly as they can help reduce cholesterol levels. Sources include olive oil, rapeseed oil, avocados, hazelnuts and almonds.

Polyunsaturated Fatty Acids (PUFAs)

This chapter is, essentially, about PUFAs and how deficiencies of them in the diet can be the cause of certain health problems. These are the fats which are liquid at room temperature because they are highly unsaturated. Polyunsaturated fatty acids are classified into omega-3 or omega-6 families. The 'parent' of the omega-3 fatty acid family is alpha linolenic acid (ALA) and the 'parent' of the omega-6 fatty acid family is linoleic acid (LA). ALA and LA are considered to be essential fatty acids (EFAs) because the body is unable to synthesize them and so we must get them from our diet.

These EFAs have three main functions: metabolism and the provision of energy, the formation of cell membranes, and the synthesis of hormone-type substances (mainly prostaglandins and leukotrienes).

Omega-3 and omega-6 fatty acids are metabolically and functionally distinct; one cannot be substituted for the other. The prostaglandins produced by omega-6 fatty acids are referred to as series-1 and series-2. The prostaglandins produced by omega-3 fatty acids are referred as series-3. Series-1 and series-3 are considered the most desirable because they reduce inflammation, thin the blood and improve circulation by dilating blood vessels. They also regulate the immune system and reproductive system. Series-2 prostaglandins tend to be antagonistic to series-1 and -3: they promote blood clotting, constrict blood flow and promote inflammation. These actions, though they may not sound it, are sometimes essential, particularly during the stress response – but are required less frequently.

The omega-6 fatty acids are widely found in seeds and their oils, especially sunflower seeds, corn oil and soya oil. Omega-6 fatty acids are involved in maintaining water balance, nerve and immune function, menstrual health, and skin and cell membrane integrity. However, because they can, as mentioned, also be converted to pro-inflammatory agents (the series-2 prostaglandins), it is important that we don't overconsume them in relation to omega-3 fatty acids.

The omega-3 fatty acids are found mostly in oily fish (salmon, mackerel, anchovy, sardines, herring, fresh tuna) flaxseed (also known as linseed) oil, walnuts, hemp seeds, pumpkin seeds and green leafy vegetables. ALA is converted to eicosapentaenoic acid (EPA) and docosahexaenoic acid (DHA) and then to prostaglandins series-3. Omega-3 fatty acids are required for cognitive function, vision, coordination, immunity and growth.

The brain, retina of the eye, testis and sperm are particularly rich in DHA. EPA can block the creation of pro-inflammatory prostaglandins and is therefore an excellent anti-inflammatory agent.

So the reason you need omega-3 fatty acids is because what you want is EPA and DHA. Here's the problem: unless you eat oily fish you'll be hard pushed to get the EPA and DHA you need. Yes, certain plant foods such as flaxseed, walnuts and green leafy vegetables contain omega-3 oils, but the body has to convert these oils into EPA and DHA. It does so rather inefficiently: it is estimated that only around 3 per cent of plant-source omega-3 is converted to EPA and DHA, if that. Oily fish is a ready-made, rich source of EPA and DHA – no conversion required. Very small amounts may also be found in poultry and eggs and in the fat of cattle, depending on how they are fed. So when food packaging boasts that its contents are rich in omega-3 oil, remember that unless the product contains fish, or fish oil, you probably won't be getting any EPA or DHA, which is what you actually want.

GETTING THE BALANCE RIGHT

There is substantial evidence to suggest that humans evolved on a diet containing equal amounts of omega-3 and omega-6.[8] However, our highly processed, modern diets have tipped the ratio and we now get a staggering 15–16 times more omega-6 than omega-3.[9] Excessive omega-6 is believed to promote many modern diseases, including heart disease, cancer and inflammatory disorders such as arthritis.[10] The reason for this is the excessive production of pro-inflammatory prostaglandins and leukotrienes, which arise from a high omega-6 consumption. This results in increases in blood viscosity (stickiness), plaques, constriction of blood vessels and other inflammatory conditions such as asthma[11] and rheumatoid arthritis.[12]

Although omega-3 fatty acids increase the production of anti-inflammatory prostaglandins, high levels of omega-6 tend to suppress the metabolic pathway of omega-3 fatty acids.

FAT-EATING HISTORY

When did it all start to go wrong? Quite a long time ago – in fact, when we started farming. Agriculture began around 10,000–12,000 years ago. Before then, grains such as wheat, corn and rice, which are sources of omega-6 oils, were not part of the human diet. Now we rely so entirely on these newcomers that shortages can cause catastrophic famines in many parts of the world.

Having said that, our problems really only started around 100 or so years ago when we started using vegetable oils in food processing and cooking. Before then we still ate a diet relatively high in omega-3 oils. The last 100 years have seen an acceleration of changes to the human diet, away from the natural diet of our pre-agricultural hunter-gatherer ancestors. These ancestors would have eaten a great deal of fish, leafy greens, wild meat, berries, nuts and other foods growing in the wild, all of which were good sources of omega-3 fats. The wild meat they consumed would have contained much more omega-3 than the grain-fed, omega-6-rich meat of farmed livestock today. The same goes for eggs

– the omega-6 to omega-3 ratio depends on the diet of the bird in question. Farmed fish contains fewer omega-3 fatty acids than fish living naturally in the sea or rivers.[13] When you consider our aquatic origins, it is hardly surprising that wild food from the sea is so wonderfully compatible with the requirements of the human body. You might not see yourself as having discernible fish-like qualities, but we humans have many physical characteristics in common with aquatic mammals, such as our large brains.[14] The sea provides us with the fish and the fatty acids they contain, which brought about the development of these large brains.[15]

We know that fish is a highly nutritious food, yet despite this – and despite being an island nation situated in the middle of a huge fish pond – the majority of the UK population does not consume nearly enough fish, particularly the oily variety, and should, according to Government advisers, be encouraged to increase consumption.[16] We currently consume 59 per cent less oily fish than we did 60 years ago.

Before the advent of the Industrial Revolution, we ate copious amounts of cheap, abundant fish. The rivers were bursting with freshwater fish, which was in fact a staple of the poor, as was salted herring. The early medieval church was responsible for the introduction of Friday as fish day, as it believed that meat incited lust. Fish was promoted to help discourage any lascivious activities amongst the peasant population. The church may now have little influence over the modern diet, but the UK Food Standards Agency does advise that we should all be eating at least two portions of fish a week, one of which should be oily.

That isn't really a great deal, when you consider our dietary history. The FSA is cautious, however, not because of any of the nutritional qualities or moral values of eating fish, but because of the toxins it may contain.

WHAT LIES BENEATH

Fish is so good, there has to be a catch, as it were. Thanks to human meddling, there is, and this is where the dilemma arises: fish in the sea and in rivers is at risk of contamination from pollutants, especially dioxins and PCBs (polychlorinated biphenyls).

Dioxins and PCBs are highly persistent chemicals widely dispersed in the environment, including the sea. These are believed to be harmful if they accumulate in the body over time. They do not break down easily and are stored in the fatty tissues of animals, including fish and humans. Like mercury, a neurotoxin also found in the sea, they are readily absorbed from the gut, and once in the blood can migrate to every cell in the body.

The issue of toxicity is of particular concern to pregnant and breastfeeding women. Requirements for omega-3 increase during pregnancy, due to the development of the baby's nervous system. Because mercury accumulates up the food chain, the largest fish have the highest levels. For this reason, pregnant and breastfeeding women are advised to avoid shark, swordfish and marlin completely. However, the advice from the FSA is that women should continue to eat other, smaller fish because the health benefits outweigh the risks. At the same time no one knows what the cumulative effect of ingesting toxins from fish is, over a long period of time.

SUPPLEMENTARY BENEFITS

If this dilemma is too much for you, there remains another option: fish oil supplements. These are screened for toxins, and an FSA survey on fish oil supplements found that most contained acceptably low levels of dioxins.[17] According to the Scientific Advisory Committee on Nutrition, no adverse effects of omega-3 fatty acid supplementation have been observed in pregnant women.[18] Of course this does not mean to say that what is currently considered to be 'acceptably low levels' are harmless; we simply don't know. Adverse effects of omega-3 fatty acid supplementation are probably impossible to detect, unless they are immediate and obvious. So you take your chances. Personally I agree with the FSA that the benefits outweigh any possible harmful effects.

EFA (OMEGA-3) DEFICIENCY AND CHRONIC DISEASE

Despite the massive changes in human diet, human genes have not changed since the Neolithic, hunter-gatherer era, so the human body has not had time to adapt to these dietary mutations. Omega-3 fatty acids are just as essential today to growth and development throughout the life cycle as they were when we were running around in skins, picking berries and clubbing small animals.

Our requirements begin at conception – EPA and DHA are critical for the development of the foetal central nervous system in the womb. Most brain development occurs during foetal development (especially in the third trimester, when the brain increases four- to fivefold in weight) and immediately after birth. Fatty acids, predominantly the PUFAs and especially DHA, are highly concentrated in the brain. The human infant has a high demand for DHA in particular, for normal brain development. Yet the infant's ability to synthesize DHA is virtually negligible.

What a mother eats could make a difference to her baby's cognitive skills. In 2005, scientists in the US announced findings that women who eat oily fish when pregnant can significantly boost the brain power of their unborn child.[19] It makes sense – the brain is over 60 per cent fat, much of which is made up of fatty acids.

The evidence is mounting that, once a child is born, his or her behaviour can also, to a certain extent, be determined by diet, and in particular by omega-3 intake. For this reason, researchers reporting the results of a randomized, controlled trial in the journal *Pediatrics* stated that fatty acid supplementation may offer a safe, effective treatment option for educational and behavioural problems among children with developmental coordination disorder.[20] Omega-3 fats have been widely researched, most famously in relation to heart health. According to the Scientific Advisory Committee on Nutrition (SACN), an organization which provides independent advice to the UK Food Standards Agency and the Department of Health, there have been numerous studies confirming the heart-health benefits of fish oil.[21] What's more, these studies have shown that the greater the intake of oily fish, the greater the reduction of risk. Increased oily fish consumption, or fish oil supplementation, decreases risk of death among patients who have already suffered a heart attack.[22] Encouragingly, heart benefits are evident within a short timescale – just a few months.[23] In 2006, 13.6 per cent of men and 13.0 per cent of women in England were reported to be diagnosed with cardiovascular disease.[24]

If you've survived childhood and middle-age, and managed to maintain a healthy heart in the meantime, you still can't afford to cut back on the fish. As we get older, we all fear decline in cognitive function. It appears that one of the best ways to boost memory and brain function is by consuming oily fish: researchers in the US have discovered that eating fish at least once a week may slow down the onset of dementia.[25]

Symptoms of EFA Deficiency

On a totally fat-free diet, EFA deficiency is extremely serious and can eventually lead to death. It is therefore logical to assume that, between extreme life-threatening deficiency and optimal intake, there are varying degrees of insufficiency, ranging from mild to serious. It is also a logical assumption that any form of deficiency can manifest as a symptom. Again, severity of symptoms is directly related to the level of deficiency.

Severe deficiency may manifest as growth retardation (in children) and multiple organ impairment or degeneration in adults. What we are concerned with here, however, are the more subtle signs which may indicate a mild deficiency. You may not have chronic disease, but you can still experience the symptoms of inadequate EFA levels. We have seen how consumption levels of omega-3 in the general population have plummeted over the ages, aggravated by excessive omega-6 fatty acids. According to the SACN, the body's demand for these fatty acids is so great that it is believed that current levels of consumption are not likely to meet those needs. Another assumption that we might make, therefore, is that symptoms of mild deficiency must be rife. These symptoms include:

- **Dry skin.** This includes inflammatory skin conditions – fish oil is known to be beneficial in the treatment of inflammatory skin disorders.[26]

- **Dry eyes.** A higher ratio of omega-6 to omega-3 fatty acid consumption was found, in one study of the dietary habits of over 32,000 women, to be associated with significantly increased risk of dry eyes syndrome.[27] Dry eyes syndrome can lead to decreased functional visual acuity.[28] The fatty acid DHA is especially important in the development of the retina.

- **Premenstrual syndrome and/or menstrual pain.** Hormones are regulated by prostaglandins; placebo-controlled trial studies have demonstrated the beneficial effect of dietary supplementation with omega-3 fatty acids on symptoms of dysmenorrhoea, or period pain.[29]

- **Fatigue.** EFAs are required for metabolism and energy production. In 2005, a study was published in *Neuroendocrinology Letters* which found that, in patients with chronic fatigue syndrome, levels of omega-6 fatty acids were elevated, and the ratio between omega-3 and omega-6 was significantly lower. The omega-3/omega-6 ratio was 'significantly and negatively correlated to the severity of illness'.[30]

- **Depression and/or anxiety.** Mood disorders have been associated with diminished omega-3 fatty acid concentrations.[31] A much-publicized review of numerous studies into the effect of food on the brain, carried out by the Mental Health Foundation in the UK, concluded that low intake of omega-3 fats is linked to depression, including post-natal depression.[32]

- **Poor memory and/or concentration.** About 20 per cent of the brain is made from EFAs. No wonder, then, that deficiency of EFAs has been linked to depression, poor cognitive function, poor memory and poor concentration.[33]

Whenever I see a client whom I suspect might have EFA deficiency, I always ask certain questions. I want to know if he or she suffers from dry skin and/or eyes. I want to know about mood, memory and concentration, and (if my client is a woman of menstruating age) if she suffers from PMS and/or painful periods. I cannot stress enough how individual symptoms may be due to any number of causes; what I look for are *clusters* of symptoms. To my mind, anyone suffering from dry skin and eyes, anxiety, menstrual pain and aching joints, for example, is quite possibly experiencing EFA deficiency.

I am always surprised by how frequently young people, especially women, report the need to moisturize all over every day because of their dry skin. Many of these people describe themselves as having skin like a lizard, or fish scales.

If women complain not only of dryness but also premenstrual symptoms and menstrual pain (also known as dysmenorrhoea) my suspicions that omega-3 fatty acids are deficient are greatly heightened. Dysmenorrhoea is an extremely unpleasant experience, the severity of which can vary. The pain can be debilitating, and accompanied by vomiting, diarrhoea and fainting. These symptoms are due to the inflammatory effect caused by the release of omega-6 fatty acids and subsequent prostaglandins and leukotrienes into the uterus just before menstruation. The result is cramping and pain. I have found supplementation with fish oil to be extraordinarily effective in the treatment of this dreadful condition. I know this from personal experience as well as professional practice. Rarely have I found this treatment to be ineffective.

SO WHAT DO YOU DO?

If you are starting to suspect that EFA deficiency is creating some or all of your health problems, the next step is to look at your diet. Do you eat a lot of oily fish, nuts, seeds and dark leafy greens? Or perhaps not? Do you make all your own food, or do you find yourself depending more than perhaps you ought to on ready-made meals? Are your cupboards crammed full of processed foods? For processed foods read omega-6 fatty acids, which might be diminishing your already dwindling levels of omega-3. Do you eat a lot of bread, pasta, rice and corn-based meals?

It is relatively simple to find out whether or not you have an EFA – or, more specifically, omega-3 – deficiency. Basically, all you do is up your omega-3 intake and lower your omega-6 intake. You need to greatly increase your intake of these fatty acids, simultaneously decreasing your intake of vegetable oils, processed foods and grains. You may also benefit from taking fish oil supplements. You also need to be aware of certain foods which interfere with the metabolism of these fatty acids, and avoid them. Alcohol is notorious for its effects on fatty acid metabolism and should be drunk only in moderation. If you are indeed omega-3 deficient you can expect speedy results – usually within a week or so of making positive changes, in my experience. Obviously for menstruation problems you will have to be a bit more patient and follow the regime for a full cycle before you can expect to see results.

Foods to Add to Your Diet

- Oily fish: mackerel, sardines, herring, salmon (wild), trout (wild), whitebait, tuna (fresh or frozen, not tinned)

- Dark leafy greens: aim to have a portion of these every day. Choose spinach, rocket, greens, cabbage, watercress, lamb's lettuce and so on

- Nuts and seeds: the unsalted, unroasted variety. In particular, go for walnuts, pumpkin seeds, flaxseeds, cashews, hazelnuts, Brazils, macadamias

- Extra virgin olive oil in cooking and dressings. Butter may also be used in cooking.

Foods and Drinks to Eliminate or Reduce

- Cakes, biscuits, pastries, sweets, chocolate, etc.

- Savoury snacks, such as crisps and salted biscuits

- Alcohol

- Vegetable and seed oils in cooking – corn, sunflower, safflower oils, for example

- Takeaways, ready-meals, processed foods – these are almost always high in omega-6 fatty acids.

Case History

Alison was a very complex case. She came to me with a history of ulcerative colitis and depression. Ulcerative colitis is an inflammatory bowel disorder and is usually treated with steroids, which is what Alison had been prescribed by her GP. She was not happy taking these and wanted to reduce the dosage. When I saw Alison she was 42 and had been diagnosed with ulcerative colitis at the age of 30. Her symptoms included pain, bleeding and chronic diarrhoea. I asked her about her skin – the answer was 'dry'. She also suffered from dry eyes. She had, in the past, been treated with Prozac but at the time of her appointment with me she was taking nothing for depression. Although her diet wasn't bad, she was vegetarian, ate no fish and was 'addicted' to sweets and chocolates. She had self-prescribed aloe vera juice which she found to be helpful in reducing symptoms.

I asked Alison if she would be prepared to take fish oil supplements, despite her vegetarian diet. She said she would have no problem with this as she was desperate to get better, though she did say that actually eating fish was out of the question as it would make her nauseous. I suggested that Alison take fish oil at a high dose – 3 grams a day. I also asked her to avoid anything with added sugar. She had already eliminated alcohol.

When I saw Alison several weeks later, she reported that she had much less pain, her skin was much improved and she no longer had dry eyes. Despite these considerable improvements, what surprised her most of all was the effect on her anxiety – after a lifetime of feeling anxious and irritable, she reported that she felt strangely calm and relaxed. She said she had never felt so 'unanxious' in all her life. I asked her what she attributed this to, and she said it was definitely the fish oil.

Alison's ulcerative colitis symptoms had improved but not been eliminated. We continued to meet occasionally and eventually her diarrhoea disappeared. Rectal bleeding had greatly reduced and occurred only very infrequently. There was occasional pain, but 'nothing like before'. Alison had been able to reduce the dosage of steroids with the knowledge and agreement of her GP.

FURTHER INVESTIGATIONS

Bear in mind that inflammation can also be caused by excessive insulin production, so if you suffer from inflammatory disorders such as rheumatoid arthritis or asthma you should also look at the information provided in the Solution 2 chapter: Rebalancing Blood Sugar.

Solution 5
Reversing Oestrogen Dominance

Oestrogen dominance, also known as hyper-oestrogenism, is direct evidence that what we do to our natural environment we do to ourselves. Humanity and ecology are indivisible and, like some sort of real-time instant karma, what we inflict on our habitat comes back to us and takes up residence in our glands, organs and fat stores.

Nothing better exemplifies this, to our misfortune, than oestrogen dominance. Oestrogens are female hormones, so this condition affects mainly women, but men too are susceptible to the negative consequences of oestrogen overload. They may not be aware of it, but their reproductive functioning is being slowly eroded by an excess of female hormones, or chemical interlopers masquerading as female hormones.

This is a foreboding subject, and to my mind the most alarming of all the subjects covered in this book, not least because it is partly out of our control. It is not, however, beyond our control: with some dietary and lifestyle adjustments and some botanical assistance, we can all mount a strong defence against, and reduce our vulnerability to, oestrogen dominance.

WHAT IS OESTROGEN DOMINANCE?

Not, as the term might imply, a state of female primacy, oestrogen dominance is a term used to describe a hormonal irregularity. It is usually applied to menopausal or premenopausal women, though it is increasingly used to describe the disproportionate level of oestrogen (in relation to other hormones) in women of all ages, and even in men.

In women, excess levels of oestrogen are known to be a major cause of hormone-related disorders including endometrial cancer, breast cancer, uterine fibroids, fibrocystic breasts and cervical dysplasia. In men, it is linked to testicular and prostate cancer and reduced fertility.

The source of excess oestrogen is both internal (endogenous) and external (exogenous). External oestrogen enters the body in the form of pharmaceutical hormones and man-made chemicals which mimic natural hormones but are much harsher in their effect.

Symptoms of Oestrogen Dominance

Women of all ages, even when free of hormone-related diseases, can still experience the low-level effects of oestrogen dominance. In menopausal women oestrogen dominance arises when, during the run-up to the cessation of the menstrual cycle, progesterone levels fall dramatically. Oestrogen levels also fall, but to a much lesser degree. Such hormonal disparity can lead to the unpleasant symptoms typically associated with the menopause, such as hot flushes, night sweats and mood swings. Women who are still of menstruating age may experience premenstrual syndrome, the symptoms of which often overlap with those of the menopause and include:

- irritability

- mood swings

- depression

- poor concentration and memory

- fatigue

- bloating (oedema, or water retention) especially of the abdomen, ankles, fingers

- headache

- cravings (usually for sweet foods, such as chocolate)

- breast tenderness

- decreased sex drive

- thyroid dysfunction

- weight gain

- acne.

FEMALE HORMONES AND THE MENSTRUAL CYCLE

Oestrogen and progesterone are sex (steroid) hormones. Their starting point is cholesterol, the precursor of all sex hormones. Cholesterol is used to make pregnenolone, which is then made into either progesterone or the adrenal hormone DHEA. DHEA is converted to testosterone, whereas progesterone is converted to oestrogen and other sex hormones.

Oestrogen is the collective name for a group of hormones, namely oestrone, oestradiol and oestriol. Each has a different function. The main role of oestrogen is the development of female characteristics in puberty and the regulation of the menstrual cycle. It initiates the growth of breasts and gives girls their characteristic female form. Most oestrogen is made in the ovaries from progesterone, but after the menopause it – or, rather, oestrone – continues to be produced in fat cells, muscles, adrenal glands and skin. Oestrogens also have non-reproductive functions and are involved in bone formation, cardiovascular health and mood regulation. Progesterone is made in the ovaries from pregnenolone; small amounts are also produced by the adrenal glands of both sexes and by the testes in men.

Oestrogen and progesterone are antagonistic to each other but also work together to create balance. For example, whereas oestrogen increases body fat, progesterone helps the body burn fat for energy. Oestrogen decreases and progesterone increases sex drive.

A baby girl is born with two ovaries, and these contain millions of follicles from which eggs will mature. By puberty it is thought that the number of follicles will have reduced to around 300,000. Hundreds of eggs disappear with each ovulation. By the time there are around 10,000 eggs left, ovulation is a rare occurrence.

A normal menstrual cycle lasts about 28 days. Day 1 is the first day of menstruation. During the first half of the menstrual cycle, oestrogen is the dominant hormone. Follicle-stimulating hormone (FSH), made in the anterior pituitary gland, stimulates the ovary to make oestrogen. Oestrogen in turn stimulates the build-up of blood and tissue in the uterus, in order to nourish the potential embryo. At the same time, the ovarian follicles of both ovaries are developing eggs.

Around day 12, oestrogen levels (primarily oestradiol) peak and gradually decline just as the follicle matures. Ovulation –

triggered by the rise of a hormone called luteinizing hormone – occurs around day 14 when an egg is released from one of the ovaries and moves to the outer surface of the ovary. During ovulation, oestrogen brings about changes in vaginal mucus, making it more hospitable to sperm. The follicle bursts and the egg is released into the fallopian tube, down which it travels to the uterus.

The empty follicle becomes the *corpus luteum*, which is the site of progesterone production. Progesterone is the dominant hormone during the second half of the menstrual cycle. The surge of progesterone inhibits ovulation in the other ovary. It prepares the uterine lining for fertilization and prevents it from being shed. If fertilization does occur, progesterone production increases in order to maintain the lining of the uterus and preserve the embryo. As the pregnancy progresses, the job of producing progesterone is taken over by the placenta. If fertilization does not occur, after 10 to 12 days following ovulation both oestrogen and progesterone levels fall abruptly, triggering menstruation and the start of a new cycle. Blood and uterine tissue are shed.

GLITCHES IN THE SYSTEM
Premenstrual Syndrome

As we have seen, progesterone is the dominant hormone following ovulation and preceding menstruation. Or it should be; if oestrogen levels are excessive at this stage, the action of progesterone may be blocked. This gives rise to symptoms associated with premenstrual syndrome.

For such a commonplace condition (the NHS website claims that PMS affects almost all women of child-bearing age) it is remarkable that its cause remains a mystery. According to the NHS, although the cause of PMS is unknown, it is thought to be linked to changes in hormonal status during the menstrual cycle. However that view is contrary to that of many experts, who do not believe the cause of the problem to be hormonal but cannot agree on an alternative hypothesis. In 1983, Dr Guy Abraham, professor of gynaecology and obstetrics, published a paper in the *Journal of Reproductive Medicine* categorizing what he believed to be the different types of PMS: type A (aggression), type C (carbohydrate craving), type D (depression) and type H (hydration).[1] Types A and H he attributed to oestrogen excess, type D to low oestrogen, and type C to blood-sugar imbalance. On what evidence, if any, he created these categories is not elucidated and his theory has never been proven or disproven. But, having seen countless women with symptoms of PMS, I have never known a case where symptoms did not improve enormously, or disappear altogether, just by balancing blood-sugar levels (see Solution 2 chapter) or following the dietary advice below, which is designed to help regulate oestrogen levels.

Perimenopause and the Menopause

Whether or not you manage to escape the symptoms of PMS, the menopause still looms large as the years advance. Symptoms of oestrogen dominance can be severe at this time of life.

Around the age of 45 to 50, oestrogen levels start to decline and periods may become irregular. They often become heavier (though in some cases lighter) than usual. During the ten years preceding the menopause – a time known as the perimenopause – a woman will experience anovulatory cycles, meaning she does not ovulate. Without ovulation there is no progesterone production. So, even though oestrogen output is declining, it is frequently the dominant hormone. Oestrogen production can be quite erratic, with dips and surges.

It is these surges, alongside diminished progesterone, which are responsible for many of the symptoms associated with the menopause: tender breasts, mood swings, disturbed sleep, weight gain, water retention, headaches. Uterine fibroids and fibrocystic breasts are not uncommon. Eight out of ten women are estimated to experience symptoms of some kind, and the most cited symptoms are hot flushes and night sweats. Women may also experience symptoms associated with hypothyroidism and unstable blood sugar.

A woman is said to have arrived at the menopause when she has not had a period for 12 months. The average age for this to occur is 52.

CAUSES OF OESTROGEN DOMINANCE

Like the menstrual cycle itself, the menopause is a completely natural event. Despite the negative associations carried by the menopause, many women do not experience hot flushes or other symptoms. Like PMS, symptoms identified with the menopause suggest that all is not well.

Oestrogen drops to 40 to 60 per cent of normal levels, whilst progesterone levels can drop to nearly zero at the menopause. Oestrogen production is sufficient for other bodily functions but insufficient for fertility. This is all perfectly natural, even though doctors have been and still frequently are too keen to 'manage' the menopause with hormone replacement therapy (HRT). Opponents of oestrogen therapy have suggested that a dose of natural progesterone is all that is needed to balance things out. The original champion of natural progesterone was the late Dr John Lee, who proposed that it is progesterone deficiency which causes menopausal symptoms, rather than oestrogen deficiency as is assumed by orthodox medicine. According to John Lee, no studies have ever proven a relationship between oestrogen deficiency and menopausal symptoms.[2] He claims to have successfully treated many women suffering from menopausal and PMS symptoms with 'natural' progesterone cream made from the Mexican yam plant. Which is all well and good, except that such an approach is still predicated on the assumption that changes in hormonal status are an aberration rather than a natural part of a woman's life.

After the menopause, oestrogens continue to be synthesized in various sites including the ovaries, adrenal glands, fat cells, skin and the brain. In these tissues, especially body fat, oestrogen is created by the enzyme aromatase, which converts male hormones to oestrone. Another enzyme converts oestrone to oestradiol. The ovaries continue to produce testosterone, which is converted to oestradiol, the most dominant form of oestrogen. Women who have had a partial hysterectomy – removal of the womb only – still produce oestrogen in their ovaries. A complete hysterectomy is the removal of the uterus, fallopian tubes and ovaries. In this case, oestrogen is still produced by fat cells.

The menopause, therefore, is a natural event, and changes in hormonal status are not in themselves cause for concern. But consider these facts:

- The incidence of breast cancer, the most common cancer in the UK, is rising exponentially. Between 1982 and 2006, incidence increased by a phenomenal 51 per cent. Today, one in nine women is expected to develop breast cancer at some time in her life. Risk is age-associated: 81 per cent of cases occur in women aged 50 years or over. The highest rates are in the developed world and the lowest in Africa and

Asia. However, ethnicity offers no safeguard: women from low-risk countries who migrate to high-risk countries, for example those who move from Japan to the US, acquire the risk level of their host country within two generations.[3]

- Uterine cancer is the fourth most common cancer in women in the UK. Like breast cancer, it is primarily a cancer of the developed world, with incidence rates over four times greater than those of developing countries. The highest rates are in North America. Although the number of cases remained stable between 1975 and 1993, it increased by 29.3 per cent between 1993 and 2005. Like breast cancer, risk is age-associated: 93 per cent of uterine cancer cases are diagnosed in women aged 50 years or over.[4]

- Prostate cancer is the most common cancer in men. One in ten men is expected to be diagnosed with the disease. Risk is age-related: three-quarters of cases occur in men over 65. The highest rates occur in North America and the lowest rates in Asian countries.[5] Having said that, screening rates are higher in North America, and screening is a fairly new tool. Even so, UK rates increased by almost 40 per cent between 1997 and 2006.[6]

- Testicular cancer is relatively rare, being responsible for 1–2 per cent of all male cancers. Unlike other hormone-related cancers, it occurs most commonly in young and middle-aged men. However, incidence is rising and those most at risk are white Caucasians in industrialized countries. Over the last 40 years there have been large increases in testicular cancer, with average increases of 1–6 per cent per year. In Great Britain the annual number of new cases more than doubled between 1975 and 2006.[7]

What do these cancers have in common?

1. They are rapidly increasing in incidence.

2. They mostly affect industrialized, Western countries.

3. They are all oestrogen-dependent. Hormone-related cancers are the most extreme expression of oestrogen dominance.

These three basic facts are incredibly revealing. Most specifically they tell us that the cause of these cancers is not predominantly genetic. Although women who carry faulty genes have a higher chance of developing a hormone-related cancer, genetic predisposition is low. For example, fewer than 5 per cent of all breast cancer cases are due to genetic defects.[8] These cancers are oestrogen-related, but if oestrogen is a natural hormone, what's going wrong?

There are several answers to this question, and they relate to three issues: natural oestrogen secretion and excretion, synthetic oestrogen, and environmental oestrogens. These are discussed below under three headings: lifestyle factors, pharmaceuticals and environmental factors.

Lifestyle Factors

Obesity

It is well documented that excessive oestrogen levels are linked to obesity, and obesity is linked to hormone-related cancers. The oestrogen–obesity link arises because the more body fat – adipose tissue – you have, the more oestrogen (oestrone) you make, through the activity of the enzyme aromatase. Excessive aromatase is therefore associated with oestrogen-related conditions.[9] Whereas body fat was once regarded as merely a repository of surplus calories, we know now that it is much more active than that – indeed, body fat is now recognized as the largest endocrine organ in the body.[10] After the menopause, fat cells are the main site of oestrogen production.

Diet

The liver is the organ which processes oestrogen, toxins and other redundant substances in order that they may be expelled from the body. Because most toxins are fat-soluble and hard to excrete, one of the liver's functions is to make them more water-soluble. It does this in two phases.

Phase 1 is carried out by a group of enzymes known as cytochrome P450 – enzymes whose job it is to biotransform toxins in preparation for phase 2.

In phase 2, fat-soluble substances are converted to water-soluble forms so they may be eliminated from the body. Therefore, efficient excretion of oestrogen – and therefore adequate liver function – is essential in order to avoid the detrimental effects of oestrogen overload. If the P450 detox system is overburdened, it becomes less efficient.

One sure way to overburden the liver is through alcohol consumption. Excessive alcohol consumption is associated with higher circulating oestrogen levels, and for this reason is linked to increased risk of breast cancer. This has been the finding of a number of studies, of which probably the best known was published in the American Journal of Epidemiology in 2007.[11] Interestingly, this association was found with various types of alcoholic beverage, but not red wine. Daily consumption of 10g of alcohol, which is the equivalent of about three-quarters to one alcoholic drink, was associated with a 9 per cent increase in the risk of invasive breast cancer. The more alcohol, the greater the risk: 30g/day was associated with a 43 per cent increase in risk.

A combination of high alcohol consumption with certain dietary habits is likely to increase that risk. Oestrogen is known to be excreted by dietary fibre, and without sufficient fibre there is the risk of reabsorption of old oestrogen from the intestines. When researchers evaluated the relationship of alcohol and dietary fibre intake with circulating sex hormone levels among premenopausal women, it was found that alcohol increased, and fibre-rich foods decreased, the levels of circulating sex hormones.[12]

There are other dietary offenders. Sugar and refined carbohydrates are prime suspects when it comes to hormone-altering activities. They are implicated in so many diseases, largely because they cause a sudden rise in blood-insulin levels (see Solution 2 chapter). Insulin is a growth factor, and high insulin is known to increase the risk of postmenopausal breast cancer.[13] Excess circulating insulin stimulates the ovaries to produce male hormones, and this can inhibit ovulation. Lack of ovulation means lack of progesterone, which in turn means unopposed oestrogen. High insulin levels also promote greater abdominal fat, which means more oestrogen production in fat cells.

Body fat and dietary fat are not the same thing. As we have seen, high levels of body fat are known to increase circulating oestrogen, but it is not clear to what extent, if any, eating fatty foods increases oestrogen levels. A review of the research on the subject found that there is limited evidence available to evaluate whether dietary fat alters circulating oestrogen levels.[14] Having said that, sources of dietary fat are more likely to have significant levels of xenoestrogens – chemicals which mimic oestrogen and are much more pernicious than natural oestrogen (see page 93).

This suggests that it may be what is *added* to dietary fat, rather than the fat *per se*, that affects oestrogen levels.

Exercise

Exercise has been found to reduce circulating oestrogen levels in postmenopausal women,[15] but it is not clear whether this effect is due to exercise itself or accompanying reductions in body fat. Oestrogen, in one study of premenopausal women who were not obese, was not found to be significantly altered by exercise.[16] This suggests that it is quite possible that body fat reduction is indeed the key to lowered oestrogen, though this area clearly still needs to be researched further.

Pharmaceuticals

The birth control pill (oral contraceptives) and HRT are both major sources of exogenous (external) oestrogens.

In order to make synthetic hormones, the molecular structure of natural oestrogen is altered so that it may be patented by its manufacturer. This makes it more potent than natural oestrogen. Hormones produced naturally by the body follow metabolic pathways governed by enzymes. Synthetic hormones, such as those which make up HRT and the contraceptive pill, do not have the same molecular structure as natural hormones and do not respond to enzymes in the same way. Natural hormones ebb and flow harmoniously to maintain homeostasis, whereas chemical hormones are not easily eliminated by the body. They also connect more readily to what are termed 'oestrogen-receptor sites' – docking stations – on cells, competing with and usurping natural hormones.

The history of the use of synthetic hormones to deal with 'women's problems' is a cautionary tale. Between 1948 and 1971 a drug called diethylstilbestrol (DES) was given to women in the US to regulate menstruation. It was also given to pregnant women to prevent premature labour and miscarriage, and incorporated into the contraceptive pill. DES was hailed as a wonder drug and was even used extensively in beef cattle feed to fatten them up more quickly, as it stimulated fat accumulation. It was later found to be linked to the development of cancer in the children of women who had taken DES during pregnancy – specifically vaginal, cervical and testicular cancer.

DES was part of the wave of techno-enthusiasm that swept the developed world after the Second World War. Advertisements in publications such as the *Journal of Obstetrics and Gynecology* boasted that DES was suitable for 'ALL pregnancies' and that it produced 'bigger and stronger babies'.[17] It was also regarded as a panacea for every kind of conceivable menopausal symptom. Its legacy was devastating but took years to be uncovered – symptoms were not immediately obvious and children born to mothers who had taken DES during pregnancy showed no outward sign of malformation. It is usually the case that the longer the time lapse between cause and effect, the longer it takes to identify that cause. To add irony to tragedy, it turned out that the drug did nothing to prevent miscarriages, premature births or stillbirths, and was later found to significantly increase incidence of those outcomes.[18]

Birth Control Pill

The combined oral contraceptive pill contains synthetic oestrogens and progesterone (progestogen). It prevents conception by inhibiting ovulation, thickening the mucus in the neck of the womb (making it more hostile to sperm) and thinning the lining of the womb to reduce the chance of a fertilized egg implanting itself.

Apart from the rather alarming, albeit small, increased risk of deep vein thrombosis, pulmonary embolus (clot in the lung), stroke, heart attack and breast cancer, many of the side effects associated with the Pill are similar to those associated with HRT, and include:

- breast tenderness and breast enlargement

- depression

- fluid retention

- headache

- migraine

- reduced libido

- weight gain.

Hormone Replacement Therapy (HRT)

This was first introduced to women in the 1950s as oestrogen replacement therapy (ERT) and sold to women on the premise that it would save them from becoming old hags by keeping them 'feminine forever'. That was the title of a book by Dr Robert A Wilson, a highly influential proponent of ERT. His book was a huge hit with the press. Before you knew it, the menopause was a disease rather than a stage of life. This marketing triumph met no resistance even though, on reflection, it was on a par with regarding puberty and all its traumas as an abnormality which needed to be managed pharmaceutically.

Very little research had been carried out into the safety of ERT, but even so any suggestions of serious side effects were dismissed outright. But all sorts of problems were beginning to emerge, not least of all uterine cancer. It was thought that 'unopposed' oestrogen was the cause of uterine cancer, so synthetic progesterone was added to ERT, which then became HRT.

HRT is undoubtedly effective at controlling the symptoms commonly associated with the menopause. However, it still comes with risks. The Medicines and Healthcare Products Regulatory Agency (MHRA) is the UK Government agency responsible for ensuring the safety of medicines. In their September 2007 *Hormone-replacement therapy: safety update*, the MHRA advises that HRT is associated not only with cardiovascular disease but also increased risk of stroke, thrombosis, breast cancer and ovarian cancer.[19]

Risks aside, there are also unpleasant side effects associated with HRT, including:

- fluid retention

- bloating

- breast tenderness or swelling

- nausea

- leg cramps

- headaches.

Environmental Factors

In the US, beef cattle are still routinely injected with synthetic oestrogen to fatten them up. Luckily for us in the UK, the use of oestrogen as a growth-enhancer for cattle is prohibited by the EU, as is, for the time being, the import of American beef (much to the annoyance of the Americans). But there are other ways for synthetic oestrogens to insinuate themselves into our bodies. It has been proposed that sewage-treatment water is a potential medium for the mass distribution of synthetic oestrogens, not to mention environmental oestrogens. Whether or not oestrogens from the contraceptive pill and HRT end up in our drinking water has been much debated but not clearly established. The water supply in England and Wales is regulated by the Drinking Water Inspectorate, which claims that it is 'confident that ordinary water treatment is effective at removing these substances'.[20] We can only hope that they are correct in their assessment. In the meantime we should perhaps concern ourselves more urgently with the risks posed by other sources of chemical hormones – xenoestrogens.

Xenoestrogens (Endocrine-disrupting Chemicals)

Undoubtedly, most egregious of all the oestrogens are the xenoestrogens. These are not actually oestrogens at all; these are toxic chemicals which make their way into the environment and which have oestrogen-like activity. Like pharmaceutical hormones, they are much more potent than the natural original. These aggressive interlopers compete with natural oestrogen and are able to lock onto the hormone receptor of a cell, switching on hormonal activity. They are found specifically in petrochemical derivatives such as plastics, pesticides, herbicides and dioxins, polychlorinated biphenyls (PCBs), refrigerants, industrial solvents, detergents and toiletries – soaps, make-up, perfume and other cosmetics.

These chemical counterfeits disrupt delicate hormone systems not just in humans but also in wildlife. PCBs – found in the sea and water supplies – accumulate up the food chain, so the larger the fish, the greater the concentration. They make their way to the fatty tissue of the fish and act on the endocrine system, where they create defective sexual organs and impair fertility as well as giving rise to behavioural abnormalities. They are considered to be 'persistent' products in that they resist the natural processes of recycling and excretion that would ordinarily render them harmless.[21]

Although this chapter addresses the symptoms of oestrogen dominance common to women, it is worth mentioning that, in men, falling sperm count is increasingly believed to be due to environmental xenoestrogens. In 1992, the *British Medical Journal* published a Danish paper which systematically reviewed studies involving almost 15,000 men from 20 countries across the world, from North America to Africa.[22] The researchers found that the average male sperm count had dropped 45 per cent, from an average of 113 million per millilitre of semen in 1940 to just 66 million per millilitre in 1990. Numerous studies since then have found similar results, citing environmental toxins as a likely culprit.

These xenoestrogens are inescapable because we live in a world dependent upon petrochemical derivatives. We may only be exposed to minute amounts of xenoestrogens from any one source, but we are exposed to myriad sources, every day of our lives. Their omnipresence means that we are susceptible to the effects of oestrogen from conception.

Plastics

Plastics are probably the most ubiquitous source of hormone disrupters. This is the age of plastic; plastic is to the consumer society of the modern age what stone was to the hunter-gatherer of the Stone Age. We have become, in less than 100 years, totally in thrall to this material.

Plastics do not degrade readily in the environment, where they tend to linger almost indefinitely. Ditto their presence in the human body. They are a significant source of xenoestrogens commonly used to make food containers, packaging and drinks bottles. This includes mineral-water bottles. When scientists analysed the contents of commercial, bottled mineral water, they found widespread contamination with xenoestrogens from the plastic. The researchers concluded, in their report, that 'a broader range of foodstuff may be contaminated with endocrine disruptors when packed with plastic'.[23]

Another oestrogen mimic, bisphenol-A, leaches from a different kind of plastic, polycarbonate. Bisphenol-A is an oestrogenic compound found in a wide range of products, including dental materials and food containers. Heating plastics, for example in a microwave oven, releases these xenoestrogens into the food and drink they contain. Bisphenol-A has been detected in canned food and human saliva. Somewhat disturbingly, it is similar in structure and behaviour to DES (the drug diethylstilbestrol, see page 90).[24]

Nonylphenols

Another source of xenoestrogens are nonylphenol ethoxylates (NPEs). NPEs are a group of man-made chemicals, primarily used in the manufacture of cleaning products such as detergents. Because of their versatility they are used in a variety of materials, including plastics, rubber (including condoms), pesticides, pharmaceuticals, cosmetics and paints.

NPEs and their primary degradation products, nonylphenols, can be highly toxic to wildlife, especially to certain water-dwelling organisms. Like other chemical hormone mimics, they are persistent and cumulative in living organisms. They easily enter the body, either through inhalation, ingestion of contaminated food or water, or through the skin. They are not effectively broken down in sewage-treatment plants.

Parabens

These chemicals are found in many deodorants, cosmetic products (including moisturizers) and toothpaste, where they function as a preservative. Evidence published in 2004 in the *Journal of Applied Toxicology* indicates that these chemicals can be detected in human breast tumours.[25] Four years later, the same authors published an update of reviews which confirmed the presence of parabens in human body tissues as detected in urine samples. In their report they called for a detailed evaluation of the ability of parabens and other oestrogenic chemicals to increase female breast cancer incidence and interfere with male reproductive functions.[26]

Pesticides

Xenostrogens are fat-soluble and, consequently, a major source of these chemicals is dietary – fat, to be precise. Animal fats do not by their nature contain these chemicals, but much of what an animal eats has been treated with pesticides. Therefore, when we ingest animal fats in the form of dairy foods and meat, we accumulate these non-biodegradable chemicals and store them in our own fat. The same goes for the pesticide residues found on the fruits and vegetables that we consume.

In 1939 the first main pesticide came into use – the organochlorine DDT. Although DDT is now banned, its invention was at the time on a par with the wheel. Its creation sat well with the post-war optimism which defined the 1950s and regarded science and intensive farming as the gateway to the future. Crops were sprayed in a prophylactic manner: the more, the merrier. The safety of these chemicals was never seriously questioned, and the role of insects and bacteria in maintaining delicate ecosystems was relatively unknown.

We know now how devastating the oestrogenic effects of pesticides can be on wildlife. A large body of evidence has accumulated linking specific conditions to endocrine-disrupting pesticides in wildlife and humans, and around 127 endocrine-disrupting pesticides have been identified.[27] Food produce is regularly monitored for traces of pesticide residues by the Pesticide Residues Committee. Maximum permitted residue levels (MRLs) have been established and, although the majority of crops are found to have less than the MRL, it is common for residues above the permitted level to be detected on some crops. These excesses may well be safe, as a one-off. But what we cannot be so sure about is the 'cocktail effect' of regular ingestion of pesticides from food sources, however minimal the level may be. There are 311 licensed pesticides in use in the UK, and around 31,000 tonnes of pesticide are applied to UK crops every year, which is quite a cocktail.

PLANT PROTECTION

This section will, I hope, restore to you the will to live, which I fear has now evaporated. There are many dietary tactics for the despondent. We know that cases and death rates of breast cancer – one of the most extreme expressions of oestrogen dominance – are markedly lower in southern as opposed to northern Europe.[28] This suggests that oestrogen dominance is less pervasive in the south, so the question is, why? When researchers assessed the effect of a 'Mediterranean' diet on oestrogen levels of healthy postmenopausal women, it was found that after six months of adopting a high plant-based diet, women who took part in the intervention were found to have a significant – over 40 per cent – decrease in total oestrogen levels.[29] This dietary intervention involved 115 women (106 completed the study) who followed a traditional Sicilian diet based on:

- pumpkin, sesame and sunflower seeds

- almonds, pistachios

- garlic, onions, fennel, carrot

- beans: chickpeas, lupins, broad beans, peas, lentils

- cauliflower and broccoli

- tomato

- extra virgin olive oil

- olives

- red grapes, figs, pomegranate, berries

- orange juice

- red chilli pepper

- red wine

- sardines, mackerel, tuna, swordfish and anchovy

- wholegrains.

A control group of women, who for the same period of time made no modifications to their usual diet, showed no significant change in oestrogen levels.

What is it about such a diet that it is able to modulate hormone expression? The Mediterranean diet's USP is that it is rich in plant foods which help reduce the body's overall load of excess oestrogens. They do this by either promoting the excretion of old oestrogen (oestrogen excreters) or preventing dangerous oestrogens from latching onto oestrogen-receptor sites (oestrogen inhibitors). These two types of plant activity are described below.

Oestrogen Excreters

Indole-3-carbinol

Indole-3-carbinol is a natural chemical which actively promotes the metabolism and breakdown of oestrogen in the liver via enzymes involved in the two phases of detoxification. The cruciferous (cabbage) family of vegetables contains this magic ingredient. These vegetables include broccoli, spring greens, cauliflower, Brussels sprouts, kale and cabbage. Other members of the cruciferous family include asparagus, spinach, celery, beetroot, cress, watercress, mustard, radish and turnip. They also contain another magic ingredient: glucosinolates. These are sulphur-containing glycosides which are metabolized by bacteria in the gut into isothiocynates, believed to be powerful anti-carcinogens.

Limonene

This is a chemical found in the oils of citrus fruits which promotes the detoxification of excessive oestrogen by the liver by inducing phase 1 and phase 2 enzymes. Limonene is found in lemons, oranges, grapefruit, tangerine, satsumas, kumquats and clementines.

Fibre

A high intake of dietary fibre has been found to be significantly associated with low circulating levels of oestradiol. Old oestrogen is disposed of via the liver, bile and finally the bowel. Fibre in the digestive tract binds to oestrogen and holds onto it for elimination. Without sufficient fibre in the diet, the oestrogen may be reabsorbed from the gut and back into the bloodstream. The Mediterranean diet contains a veritable glut of quality fibre: fruits, vegetables, beans, lentils, nuts and seeds.

Oestrogen Inhibitors

These are plant compounds with oestrogen-like activity, usually known as phytoestrogens. They are weaker than 'real' oestrogens but compete with them for attachment to receptor sites throughout the body.

There are four main types of phytoestrogens:

1. isoflavones (including genistein and daidzein) – legumes (peas, beans and lentils), especially soya beans, are a rich source of isoflavones

2. coumestrol – the best sources of coumestrol are legumes, and in particular soyabean sprouts

3. lignans – the main source of lignans are flaxseed (also known as linseeds), wholegrain bread, vegetables (especially squash) and tea

4. stilbenes– the main source of stilbenes are peanuts and resveratrol, a substance found in red wine. The longer the fermentation period of wine-making, the greater the level of resveratrol.

> **Legumes**
>
> peas – all types, including snap, snow, black-eyed
>
> beans – string, French, runner, broad, soya, fava, kidney, pinto, butter, haricot, cannellini, borlotti, adzuki beans, chickpeas
>
> lentils – green, brown, red, black, puy

There has been much debate over whether plant oestrogens are healthful or harmful to human health. If man-made, chemical oestrogens are so noxious, how do we know that plant oestrogens are beneficial? Chemical mimics are hazardous because they can persist in the body for years. They are extremely difficult to shift, being fat-soluble, cumulative and non-biodegradable. Plant oestrogens, on the other hand, closely resemble natural human oestrogen and are quickly metabolized and easily eliminated. After ingestion through diet, they are metabolized by intestinal bacteria, absorbed, reconjugated by the liver, circulated in the blood and then excreted in the urine.[30] Phytoestrogens have both oestrogenic and anti-oestrogenic properties, helping to block stronger, more toxic oestrogens from latching onto oestrogen-receptors. In large amounts they actually displace oestradiol from receptor sites. As well as occupying oestrogen-receptors, phytoestrogens, especially isoflavones, inhibit the action of the enzyme aromatase, which, as already mentioned, promotes the synthesis of oestrogen.[31] It is their dual capacity to exert both oestrogenic and anti-oestrogenic activity which has led to confusion over whether or not phytoestrogens are benign. In the 1940s it was first observed that sheep grazing on pastures rich in red clover, which has high amounts of isoflavones, developed fertility problems and frequent miscarriage. However, in humans, a regular intake of phytoestrogens appears to be protective. This is evidenced by Japan, for example, where the incidence of breast cancer is approximately one-third that of Western countries. The Japanese have a high intake of dietary phytoestrogens, and soya is a staple of the Japanese diet.[32]

There is a plethora of research on the effects of regular soya intake on the endocrine system, and there is no doubt that it appears to be beneficial. The real cause for concern may be the effect of feeding babies exclusively on soya milk – rather like cattle feeding exclusively on clover. Perhaps if adult humans grazed all day on clover, or even tofu, they too might develop fertility problems – we just don't know, but such a diet is intuitively wrong. Yet, as a regular part of a mixed and varied human diet, soya, in the form of tofu or miso, for example, appears to be only beneficial. I am no fan of soya from a culinary perspective (to me it is the epitome of bland) but, given the choice between soya oestrogens and xenoestrogens, I know which I would rather have latching onto my receptors.

Gut Bacteria

There is evidence that, in order to be of any use, phytoestrogens need to be metabolized by gut bacteria in order to be absorbed.[33] These gut bacteria are essential for health overall, and you can read all about them in the Solution 7 chapter.

HERBALS

If you have more advanced symptoms of oestrogen dominance, such as fibroids or polycystic ovaries, I recommend you consider seeing a medical herbalist as there are many fantastic herbal extracts which are known to help balance sex hormones. But for ordinary, run-of-the-mill symptoms associated with PMS and the menopause, I can't recommend the herbal extract *Agnus castus* enough. Also known as chasteberry, this plant has been shown to exhibit 'significant competitive binding' to oestrogen-receptors.[34] In a study of over 200 women with moderate to severe PMS, *Agnus castus* was found to be a safe, well-tolerated and effective treatment. [35]

A BRIEF GUIDE TO STABILIZING YOUR OESTROGEN LEVELS

What to eat (and drink)	High-fibre diet – see the Mediterranean diet (page 98)	Oestrogen is known to be excreted by dietary fibre, and without sufficient fibre there is the risk of reabsorption of old oestrogen.
	Drink filtered water whenever possible. Best of all, install a water filter under the sink.	Bottled mineral water has been found to be contaminated with xenoestrogens.
	Eat organic food wherever possible, especially food containing fats.	The use of pesticides is severely restricted in organic farming – a handful only are allowed when absolutely essential.
	Eat plenty of phytoestrogen-rich foods.	Phytoestrogens are weak, plant oestrogens which help regulate oestrogens in the body.

What not to eat (or drink)	Alcohol	Alcohol consumption is associated with higher circulating oestrogen levels. If you do drink, stick with moderate quantities of red wine as it contains the phytoestrogen resveratrol.
	Sugar and refined carbohydrates	These raise insulin levels, and insulin increases the risk of postmenopausal breast cancer, and also raises body fat and oestrogen levels.
Dos and Don'ts	Lose weight if you are overweight or obese.	The more body fat – adipose tissue – you have, the more oestrogen (oestrone) you make, through the activity of the enzyme aromatase.
	Use natural cosmetics and toiletries if you can't do without them. Check labels for parabens.	Parabens are xenoestrogens detectable in human tissue.
	Establish good intestinal bacteria (see Solution 7 chapter).	Intestinal bacteria are need to metabolize plant oestrogens.

Dos and Don'ts	Do not use the contraceptive pill or HRT, if at all possible.	Both are major sources of synthetic oestrogens.
	Don't heat food in plastic containers.	Heating plastics increases leaching of xenoestrogens into food.
	Don't wrap fatty foods in cling film.	Cling film is a source of xenoestrogens which can leach easily into fatty foods.

Case History

Caitlin was 30 when she first came to see me. She had three main health problems she wanted to address: irregular periods, mood swings, and being overweight. On questioning, it turned out she had a fair few other symptoms. These included low energy, poor concentration, premenstrual syndrome, headaches, insomnia, anxiety and night sweats. Her diet wasn't too bad, in that she ate lots of fruit, but she also ate lots of sugary foods and drank fizzy drinks. She had previously been on the Pill for four years and, although had not taken it for two years, her periods had never normalized since stopping. Her diet was also extraordinarily high in wheat – endless bread and pasta. My first thought was oestrogen dominance. To start with, I asked Caitlin to remove the sugar component of her diet and to increase phytoestrogens, including tofu and lots of green leafy cruciferous vegetables. I asked her to focus especially on eating lots more beans and lentils, live yoghurt (for the friendly bacteria), onions and garlic (believed to help with the detoxification pathways of the liver) and citrus fruits. I asked her to cut down on her wheat intake, mainly in order to make room for beans and lentils. She hardly drank any alcohol so there was no need to advise on this. In the way of supplements, I gave her a good basic multivitamin and -mineral supplement, with all the main B vitamins, and some fish oil, as fish oil helps regulate hormone production.

The second time I saw Caitlin, about five weeks later, she reported that a number of her symptoms had improved – energy levels were up considerably and she was sleeping well right through the night. She had still had some PMS symptoms, namely irritability and headaches, but these were much reduced. She had also lost about 7 lb in weight. This time I added *Agnus castus* to her programme.

By the time I saw her a third time, about six weeks after her second appointment, she reported that all PMS symptoms had completely vanished and she had lost 14 lb in total.

OTHER THERAPIES

Herbal medicine is excellent if your symptoms are particularly severe, or if you have fibroids, endometriosis, PCOS, etc.

FURTHER INVESTIGATIONS

If you suspect you have oestrogen dominance you should definitely have a look at Solutions 7 and 8, as gut bacteria, as we have seen, play a major role in the metabolism of phytoestrogens. A leaky gut can overburden the liver, making it all the harder to excrete excessive oestrogen.

Make sure you also read the Solution 2 chapter: Rebalancing Blood Sugar. Blood-sugar imbalance can severely aggravate the symptoms of premenstrual syndrome, and high insulin levels can result in raised oestrogen levels.

Solution 6

Correcting Mild
Hypothyroidism

Hypothyroidism, or underactive thyroid, is a tricky subject. Its symptoms are wide-ranging and non-specific, and turn up in all sorts of other health problems. Trickier still is the subject of *mild* hypothyroidism. For some in the medical establishment, mild hypothyroidism is simply not a problem because it falls outside the diagnosis radar, as defined by blood tests. However, that opinion is changing, as more doctors and researchers are beginning to question the definition of 'normal' with regard to the reference ranges set by laboratories to assess the level of thyroid hormones in the blood.

In the meantime, and until there is a shift in the received wisdom on the subject, the best you can do is be as well informed as possible on the workings of the thyroid gland. This chapter is a guide to those of you who feel you might have mild, or sub-clinical, hypothyroidism; those of you who find yourself in the situation of having had the tests and been given the all-clear, whilst experiencing the symptoms of a condition you technically don't have. It is an unfortunate fact that it is usually only when symptoms become bad enough to show up on blood tests that any help becomes available.

First, a bit of background on what the thyroid does, and how it can go wrong.

ANATOMY OF A GLAND

The thyroid is a gland at the front of the neck, shaped rather like a butterfly and consisting of two lobes, one on either side of the wind-pipe and joined by tissue called the isthmus. It governs metabolism in virtually every cell of the body and is responsible for your overall metabolic rate – in other words, the speed at which you burn food for fuel.

Hormones are secreted by the thyroid as part of a process of hormone production which begins in a section of the brain called the hypothalamus. The hypothalamus produces a hormone called thyrotrophin-releasing hormone (TRH). TRH travels to the pituitary, a gland in the brain, where it stimulates the release of thyroid-stimulating hormone (TSH). TSH does exactly as its name suggests: it stimulates the thyroid to produce hormones. Two hormones, to be precise. These are thyroxine (aka T4 because it contains four atoms of iodine) and triiodothyronine (aka T3 because it contains three atoms of iodine). Thyroid hormone is the term used to describe both these hormones together. T4 is converted to T3, its active form, in the thyroid but also in other parts of the body, including the liver and the brain. However, this conversion takes place only if the body is up to the job. An inability to convert T4 to T3 can cause problems, but more of this later. The pituitary gland is a sensitive feedback device: it detects levels of circulating thyroid hormone and adjusts output accordingly. As thyroid hormone levels in the blood decline, TSH levels increase. As thyroid hormone increases, TSH decreases.

Almost all of the thyroid hormone in your blood is transported around by proteins. But a very small amount – 0.03 per cent – is not attached to proteins and is described as being 'free'. It is only this free thyroid hormone which can enter the body's cells and be of any use. It is extraordinary but true that, to date, no one knows what the point is of all that protein-bound thyroid hormone in the body.

What the Thyroid Does

The hormones produced by the thyroid stimulate metabolism and are responsible for your basal metabolic rate (BMR) by regulating the speed at which cellular activity is carried out. Your BMR is the rate at which you metabolize nutrients when at rest. Metabolic activity creates heat, so the thyroid is also responsible for maintaining body temperature. That is why coldness is a symptom of hypothyroidism. Thyroid hormone stimulates the metabolism of protein in muscles, as well as carbohydrates and fats for energy. So if you don't produce enough thyroid hormone, you may find you put on weight rather too easily.

All organs depend on the thyroid gland: the heart relies on thyroid hormone to pump blood, lungs need it for respiration, the intestinal tract for the transition of food. Bones require thyroid hormone for growth. It stimulates brain activity, which is why excessive amounts can cause overanxiety and too little can result in mental apathy.

THYROID DISEASE

Thyroid disease is the name given to any thyroid condition. Women are much more likely to have some sort of thyroid disorder than men. It is also more common in people over the age of 35, and often runs in families.

It is impossible to say just how common thyroid disease is, because the answer depends on whom you ask. According to Dr Barry Durrant-Peatfield, author of *Your Thyroid and How to Keep it Healthy*, estimates – made by physicians specializing in hypothyroidism – range from 10 per cent of the population to 80 per cent.[1] Those figures are much higher than official estimates, which state that about 1.9 per cent of women and 0.1 per cent of men in the UK will develop hypothyroidism at some point in their lives. About 2 per cent of women and 0.2 per cent of men will develop *hyper*thyroidism – overactive thyroid – at some point in their lives.

You are more at risk of developing thyroid disease if:

- there is a family history of the condition

- you are pregnant

- you have coeliac disease or any other autoimmune disorder (see below)

- you have been exposed to radiation

- you are on certain medications which can trigger disease, notably lithium

- you have a low intake of iodine

- you are diabetic. It has been estimated that 10.8 per cent of diabetics have thyroid disease.[2]

There are several types of thyroid disease; the most common are hyperthyroidism, goitre, thyroiditis, thyroid eye disease, nodules, thyroid cancer and hypothyroidism. If you have normal thyroid activity, you are described as being *euthyroid*.

Hyperthyroidism

The opposite of hypothyroidism, with this condition the thyroid produces too much thyroid hormone rather than too little. Therefore symptoms are a direct opposite of those of hypothyroidism: everything is too fast rather than too slow.

Signs and Symptoms

* weight loss

* insomnia

* hyperactivity

* rapid heart beat

* palpitations

* diarrhoea/frequent bowel movements

* high blood pressure

* irritability

* anxiety

* dry skin or thickening of the skin

* brittle hair

* tremor

* menstrual irregularities

* feeling of 'overheating'

- bulging eyes

- 'club' nails

- visibly enlarged thyroid gland.

What Causes Hyperthyroidism?

The most common cause of hyperthyroidism is Graves' disease, which is an autoimmune disorder where the body produces thyroid-stimulation antibody (TSA) which attacks the thyroid. In response to this attack, the thyroid overproduces thyroid hormone. Graves' disease is more likely to occur if other family members have also been affected.

Treatment for Hyperthyroidism

Hyperthyroidism is usually treated with anti-thyroid drugs which suppress the production of thyroid hormone. It may also be treated with beta-blockers to calm the heart rate. In some cases part of the thyroid may be surgically removed in a procedure known as partial thyroidectomy. This can be a bit tricky as exactly the right amount needs to be removed to be effective and to avoid hypothyroidism arising from removing too much. Giving radioiodine (radioactive iodine in pill form) is another form of treatment as it reduces the gland's activity. This form of treatment is not given to children or pregnant or breastfeeding women and can only be carried out by authorized medical staff.

Goitre

This is an enlarged thyroid gland which is visible as a swelling in the neck. A goitre can be caused by either hypothyroidism or hyperthyroidism. It can also be caused by insufficient or excessive iodine intake or elevated levels of thyroid auto-antibodies. Symptoms experienced may include difficulty swallowing, chest pain and a full feeling in the throat. There may also be shortness of breath.

Thyroiditis

This is any inflammation of the thyroid, of which there are several types, including Hashimoto's thyroiditis (see page 118). The result is mild hypothyroidism or temporary Hashimoto's. There is also postpartum thyroiditis which occurs in women just after giving birth and usually resolves itself within a few months on its own.

Thyroid Eye Disease

Also known as Graves' ophthalmopathy, this is a condition which tends to affect people with Graves' disease but it can also affect those with Hashimoto's thyroiditis. The condition is characterized by upper eyelid retraction and swelling of fatty tissue behind the eye, which makes the eye appear to bulge, giving the sufferer a startled expression. Other symptoms include dry or watery eyes, itching, a feeling of grittiness, aching eyes and double vision. The condition tends to resolve itself over time without requiring any medical intervention, although in some cases this may be necessary.

Nodules

These are usually benign lumps which grow in the thyroid and are fairly common. Symptoms are similar to those of hyperthyroidism, such as weight loss and palpitations, but can also resemble hypothyroidism. There may be difficulty swallowing, pain, tenderness and a feeling of fullness in the throat.

Thyroid Cancer

Less common is thyroid cancer, where lumps growing in the thyroid are malignant and may require surgical removal of the whole gland. This is fairly uncommon and a diagnosis will be established by biopsy. Treatment may involve radioactive iodine therapy, radiation or chemotherapy but is most likely to involve surgery to remove either part of the thyroid or all of it. Survival rate for this cancer is fortunately very high.

Hypothyroidism

Also known as an underactive thyroid, this is a condition whereby the thyroid simply isn't making enough thyroid hormone. Bearing in mind that the thyroid is the gland responsible for metabolism, if it is underactive you are likely to experience symptoms of slowness and sluggishness, both physical and mental.

Signs and Symptoms

- fatigue
- dry, coarse skin
- weight gain
- feeling cold
- hair loss
- loss of outer third of eyebrows and sometimes eyelashes
- slow pulse

- constipation

- brittle nails, sometimes grooved

- changes in skin pigmentation

- water retention, puffiness (oedema)

- hoarse or husky voice

- shortness of breath

- enlarged thyroid (goitre)

- aching muscles

- apathy

- depression, including post-natal depression

- poor night vision

- menstrual irregularities/infertility

- slow heart rate

- loss of libido

What Causes Hypothyroidism?

There are many possible causes, some of which can be traced as far back as the womb. If the thyroid fails to develop properly in the unborn baby, it may be born with hypothyroidism. All babies in the UK are screened for this shortly after birth and if treated can expect to develop normally.

A major cause of hypothyroidism is autoimmune disease. An autoimmune disease is a condition whereby the body fails to recognize its own cells and instead treats them as the enemy and attacks them. Autoimmune thyroid disorders are most likely to strike during the first trimester of pregnancy or shortly after delivery.

Women generally are more prone than men. The most common autoimmune disorder to cause hypothyroidism is Hashimoto's thyroiditis. If you have an existing autoimmune disorder such as type 1 diabetes, Addison's disease or rheumatoid arthritis, your risk of developing Hashimoto's is increased. Typically with this condition TSH values are high while T3 and T4 levels are low. Hashimoto's can initially cause hyperthyroidism, but eventually leads to hypothyroidism because the thyroid's ability to produce hormones is destroyed.

Other Causes of Hypothyroidism

- Surgery. The thyroid may be fully or partially removed if there is cancer or some other condition which requires surgery. If part of the thyroid remains, hormones may still be produced but probably not in sufficient quantities.

- Medication. The best-known pharmaceutical to interfere with thyroid production is lithium – its side effects include thyroid suppression.

- Fluoride and mercury toxicity. Mercury is antagonistic to selenium, which is an essential element for thyroid health (see page 129). Fluoride is known to suppress thyroid activity and, in children, excess fluoride in drinking water has been shown to affect thyroid hormone output.[3] The jury is still out on whether or not fluoride is a cause of hypothyroidism in the general population.

- Hypothalamus and pituitary disorders. Both of these glands are involved in thyroid hormone production, so any disorder of or damage to these glands can cause hypothyroidism.

- Iodine deficiency - see below.

Iodine Deficiency

One highly significant but almost always overlooked cause of hypothyroidism is iodine deficiency. Iodine is a trace element which is a component of thyroid hormone. It is required in minute amounts – 150 micrograms (mcg) is the recommended daily intake – and is found in seafood, seaweed (where it was first discovered), dairy foods (because it is routinely added to cattle feed), some vegetables and anything which contains iodized salt.

Iodine deficiency is a major cause of hypothyroidism worldwide, with around 2 billion individuals across the globe thought to have insufficient iodine intake.[4] South Asia and sub-Saharan Africa are particularly affected. When deficiency is severe, so are the consequences, especially for growth and development. During pregnancy and early infancy, iodine deficiency can result in cretinism, which is characterized by stunted growth and mental disability, and is irreversible. Iodine deficiency is recognized by the World Health Organization as the most common preventable cause of brain damage in the world today.

The most successful and cost-effective way to prevent iodine deficiency is iodization of salt. Where this is not possible, iodine supplements may be given. The World Health Organization recommends that pregnant and breastfeeding women have a daily intake of 200 micrograms. In developing countries, iodine supplementation – in the form of iodized salt, bread or oil – has successfully prevented goitre in adults.[5]

Why Is Iodine Deficiency Such a Huge Problem Around the World?

The scale of the problem is due to the fact that most of the iodine on the planet is in the sea, not in the soil. This was not always the case. In this instance, intensive farming and human meddling cannot be held accountable for global iodine shortages. One of the main causes is glaciation during the last Ice Age, which exposed the iodine-rich layers of soil to rain, flooding and wind, which washed the iodine into the sea. Soil erosion has resulted in depletion of this crucial element everywhere, with parts of Africa, China, Russia and Asia severely iodine-deficient and all mountainous areas particularly at risk. It is not surprising, therefore, that thyroid problems are especially common in areas which were once covered by glaciers.

Iodine Deficiency in the UK

Whereas salt-iodization programmes are in place across much of the developing world, no such programme is in place in the UK. Consequently, there is very little iodized salt consumed here. That may not be such a bad thing, considering that we consume too much salt in the first place and are usually exhorted to cut down. But that still leaves the problem of potential iodine deficiency which is not being addressed. Data suggests that iodine deficiency is more common than generally believed. Although not as severe as in developing countries, mild to moderate iodine deficiency is not uncommon in European countries.[6] The more severe the deficiency, the more severe the frequency and severity of iodine-deficiency disorders.[7] A review of studies of pregnant women across Europe concluded that most women in Europe are iodine-deficient during pregnancy.[8]

There is concern that pregnant women in the UK do not have enough iodine, putting their unborn child at risk of reduced intelligence scores and impaired motor skills.[9] A study published in 2008 of 31 women in Surrey, which measured iodine concentration in urine, found that approximately 30 per cent of the women were classified as mildly to moderately iodine-deficient.[10]

Because we get most of our iodine from seafood and dairy produce, anyone who avoids these foods might be at particular risk of deficiency. Therefore vegans and vegetarians are even more vulnerable. There is a paucity of studies on iodine status in the general population, but one study of 30 vegans, published in 1998, found that 36 per cent of the males and 63 per cent of the females had lower than the recommended intake of iodine.[11]

The fact is there are no screening programmes for iodine deficiency in the UK because it is assumed that deficiency does not exist.[12] The British Nutrition Foundation states, on its website, that 'Nowadays iodine deficiency is very rare in the UK.' This is odd, because according to the Department of Health's National Diet and Nutrition Survey of Adults aged 19 to 64, in 2003, although men appeared to have an adequate intake of iodine, women aged 19–24 were found to have an average intake of 130 mcg iodine and women aged 25–34 had an average intake of 145mcg – below the recommended amount.[13]

Treatment for Hypothyroidism

The standard treatment is thyroxine, which is given as a synthetic hormone called *levothyroxine*. Thyroxine is readily converted in the body to T3, and as a result levels of TSH return to normal. It often takes a while to find the right dosage for each individual. Too much thyroid hormone replacement over a period of time can lead to symptoms of hyperthyroidism. Side effects include an increase in the risk of atrial fibrillation (irregular heart rhythm) and bone loss.

Testing for Hypothyroidism

There are various tests which your GP can arrange; those described below are the main tests in use today.

Total Thyroxine (TT4)

This test measures the amount of T4 in the blood. However, because T4 is protein-bound and therefore inactive, this is not an accurate measure of thyroid hormone. Test results can also be skewed by the fact that certain drugs, including HRT and the contraceptive pill, can produce a false high reading. Other drugs, such as steroids, can lead to a lower test reading. This test has largely been replaced by measuring free thyroxine (FT4, see below).

Free Thyroxine (FT4)

This tests the amount of free thyroxine in the blood – the thyroxine which is free to be converted to T3, the active form of thyroid hormone. Free thyroxine is not affected by drugs, although certain factors such as severe illness can influence the test outcome. However, this test does not actually indicate how much, if any, T4 is converted to T3.

Triiodothyronine (T3)

This is measured as free T3 (not protein-bound) and total T3 (attached to a protein). Although very useful, it does not measure how much T3 actually enters the cells.

Thyroid-stimulating Hormone (TSH)

This is thought to be a good measurement of either excessive or insufficient thyroid activity. A high reading indicates hypothyroidism, because the body is increasing its production and release of TSH in an effort to push up T4 levels. A separate, low T4 test result would usually confirm diagnosis. A low TSH reading suggests hyperthyroidism, because there are already high levels of T4 circulating in the blood. Again, certain conditions such as pregnancy or the presence of tumours can cause a reduction of TSH levels.

Thyroid Auto-antibody Testing

Thyroid conditions may be caused by the body failing to recognize its own tissues and therefore creating antibodies against itself. Hashimoto's thyroiditis and Graves' disease are two such conditions. The antibodies which the body creates to 'fight' itself are called auto-antibodies, and a blood test can reveal the presence of abnormal amounts of these auto-antibodies. This can cause either hyper- or hypothyroidism.

Urine Iodine Excretion

This is a very useful test, especially if you are vegetarian or vegan, or just avoid seafood and/or dairy produce. However it is not normally offered by GPs so you would probably have to arrange for it to be carried out privately (see the Resources chapter for laboratory details).

Urinary iodine excretion is believed to be a good indicator of dietary iodine intake. It also monitors excessive iodine intake.

Mild (Sub-clinical) Hypothyroidism

Sub-clinical hypothyroidism is defined as having elevated TSH levels but normal free thyroid hormone levels. If this is what your test results indicate, you are regarded as being in a pre-hypothyroid state. Sub-clinical hypothyroidism is believed to be a precursor to clinical, overt hypothyroidism. It is not considered a condition in itself, and there is ongoing debate about whether or not it should be treated. But there is another ongoing debate, and that is about whether or not the tests themselves, rather than the results, are the problem.

The Trouble with Tests

Thyroid testing is by no means conclusive – if only a simple blood test could be that simple.

The dilemma lies in the reference range – that is, the point between A and B of the test results which is considered to be 'normal'. Another difficulty is that blood tests indicate hormone levels in the *blood*, not in tissue itself, and it is thyroid hormone in tissue that counts. All too often when a test result comes back normal, the patient may be persuaded to stop worrying about his or her health problems because, according to the test results, none exists.

So, the difference between mild, or sub-clinical hypo-thyroidism and overt hypothyroidism is determined by a line on a chart mapped out by the laboratory carrying out the test. The trouble is, different laboratories set different cut-off limits of what is considered normal.

The normal range is purely arbitrary and some people believe that it is too wide, with the result that almost everyone falls into it. In the UK, the upper limit of normal for TSH may be 4.0mU/L, 5.0mU/L or even higher, depending on which laboratory performs the test. It has recently been proposed that the upper limit of 'normal' TSH in blood tests should be reduced to 3.0 or even less in order to 'catch' people with sub-clinical hypothyroidism.[14] One reason for this is that higher levels of anti-thyroid antibodies are detected in people with serum (blood) TSH levels between 3.0 and 5.0 mIU/L. The medical world has historically misinterpreted these results as 'normal'.[15] Yet patients with these results are thought more likely to go on to develop overt thyroid disease.[16]

Sub-clinical hypothyroidism is probably taken more seriously in the US, where estimates of the prevalence of this condition are

4–10 per cent of the general population and 7–26 per cent of the elderly population.[17] Sub-clinical hypothyroidism is believed by many experts to represent mild thyroid failure and, according to researchers writing in the *Journal of Clinical Endocrinology and Metabolism*, 'is a clinically important disorder that has adverse clinical consequences and that should be treated in most, if not all, cases'.[18]

People with mild hypothyroidism may experience common overt hypothyroid symptoms, especially dry skin, fatigue, poor memory, intolerance to the cold, puffy eyes, constipation and hoarseness.[19] Of three randomized, controlled studies which examined the effects of giving thyroid hormone to people with sub-clinical hypothyroidism, two reported significant improvement in symptoms.[20] Other studies have found mixed results – some positive but some with no significant improvement.[21] Clearly, more research in this area is required.

DO YOU HAVE MILD HYPOTHYROIDISM?

Here is a common scenario in my practice. A woman aged, say, between 30 and 60 comes to see me complaining of fatigue, depression, overweight and constipation. She has no get-up-and-go and feels generally apathetic. She has gone to her GP, who has arranged for an unspecified thyroid test, which has shown 'normal' results.

Me: Do you know what sort of test you had?

Client: No – just that it was a blood test.

Me: Do you have a copy of the results?

Client: No, I haven't.

Clients rarely have any idea of the details of the tests they have undergone. I always find this extraordinary and would recommend that everyone obtains a copy of the results of whatever test they have had, for future reference. Anyway, at this point I direct attention towards their main concern, which is usually but not always weight gain.

Me: Do you know why you have gained weight? What I mean is, do you feel your weight gain is justified, or is it a mystery?

Client: I don't understand it. I eat less than everyone else I know, go to the gym four days a week, but the weight's just not shifting.

Me: Do you have a history of dieting? Have you tried all sorts of extreme diets in the past?

These last two questions I consider highly significant. I have found, over and over again, that people I suspect might have mild hypothyroidism do not eat more than normal (in fact, often less) and they tell me they have been on every kind of diet for years. Severely restricting food intake is one of the best ways of guaranteeing weight gain. First you lose weight, and feel great. Then your weight reaches a plateau. Then you struggle to keep up the restricted eating, and feel depressed because you are suffering but not seeing results. Then you give up and give in to the constant hunger pangs and find you actually gain *more* weight than you lost, just by returning to your original eating habits. The fact is that drastic reduction in food intake slows down the metabolic rate – or rather, slows down the activity of the thyroid gland in an effort to retain fat stores (your Stone Age body thinks it's dealing with a famine). As calorie intake falls, so too does the level of thyroid hormone output. So you have to eat less and less to lose any weight at all or even just to maintain the same weight. You can only keep this up for so long, as every dieter will concur. This system evolved over millennia as a defence mechanism against famine and you cannot beat it. Studies have confirmed that underfeeding results in a decrease in metabolic rate.[22] More specifically, calorie restriction actually results in lowered T3 production.[23] Getting the thyroid to return to normal production, after years of calorie-restricted dieting, is not easy.

So you might be suspicious if you have any of the symptoms of overt hypothyroidism, listed above, and even more so if you are overweight but not overeating, and have a history of yo yo dieting.

WHAT TO DO IF YOU THINK YOU MIGHT HAVE MILD HYPOTHYROIDISM

First, go to your GP. If you have already had a test, but do not know what type, ask. You are entitled to know. You specifically want to know if you have had a TSH test and antibody test, as these are the most indicative. If you have not had these tests, request them. If they turn out to be positive, you will be prescribed thyroid hormone. Whatever the result, check the reference ranges of what is considered a normal reading. If the upper limit is high, i.e. 4.0mU/L or 5.0mU/L and your result is close to that borderline, remember that the limit is a contentious, arbitrary figure and some experts might consider that a positive result. Discuss this with your GP, and point out that mild hypothyroidism often progresses to overt hypothyroidism.[24]

If you prefer, you can have a test carried out privately. The *total thyroid screen* is comprehensive as it measures all thyroid hormones as well as levels of auto-antibodies: free T3, free T4, total T4 and TSH. See the Resources chapter for details of a laboratory that carries out this test. Consider the results to be for your information only: if they are positive, you should return to your GP for further discussion about what to do.

If you are vegan or have a low dairy and/or low seafood diet and do not regularly consume edible seaweeds, I suggest you have a urine iodine test. See the Resources chapter.

For your next step, you can try a useful test which you can carry out yourself at home, which is free and does not involve blood or urine samples. It is called the *basal temperature test*. This test was first described in 1945 by the famous Dr Broda Barnes, who devoted his professional life to the study of the thyroid gland. Having said that, many conventional doctors repudiate the accuracy of this test and insist that only a blood test (which is hardly free from controversy) will do. But I think that, although it is by no means conclusive, it is a very useful tool, especially if your cluster of symptoms all point towards some sort of thyroid malfunction.

The basal temperature is the body temperature when totally at rest – asleep, in fact. A low basal body temperature is thought to be indicative of an underactive thyroid. See below for details on how to do the test.

The Basal Temperature Test

Get an old-fashioned glass thermometer. Digital thermometers are not thought to be as accurate for this test.

Place it by your bed at night, having shaken it well to make sure it is at 94°F/34.4°C or below.

Take your temperature immediately on waking. Place the thermometer under your arm for a full 10 minutes and lie as still as you can.

Write down the reading.

Repeat this every morning for a couple of weeks, minimum, in order to get a good idea of your average body temperature.

Do not perform this test if you have a cold or any infection which might temporarily raise your body temperature. Drinking a fair bit of alcohol the night before can have the opposite effect, i.e. cause your body temperature to drop slightly. Women who are still of menstruating age should be sure that the second, third and fourth days of menstruation are included.

Your normal basal temperature should be between 97.8°F/36.5°C and 98.2°F/ 36.8°C. An average reading of less than this should arouse suspicion that your thyroid might be working below par.

If all your testing suggests mild hypothyroidism rather than clinical hypothyroidism, and no treatment is offered by your GP, do not despair. There are a few natural approaches which you may find beneficial. Unfortunately, dietary therapy is not always the most effective therapy – in my experience, changing a client's diet to include more of the nutrients vital to thyroid health is only effective if that client's diet is poor in the first place, and probably lacks those nutrients. The most important of these nutrients – other than iodine, which has already been discussed, are described below.

Selenium

This trace element is needed for the conversion of T4 to T3 and is present in high concentrations in the normal thyroid. Dietary selenium levels have been falling for years – as long ago as 1997 the *British Medical Journal* claimed it was 'time to act' on the worrying depletion of selenium levels in soil throughout the world, including Europe.[25] The author reported that 22 years previously, selenium intake in Britain was 60mcg/day, compared to 34mcg/day in 1997. Selenium is found in Brazil nuts (one of the richest sources), meat, fish and cereal grains.

Zinc

Is required for all hormone production, including thyroid hormone. Like selenium, it is also required for the conversion of T4 to T3. Good sources include meat, especially red meat, fish, seafood and lentils. Once absorbed in the body, it is combined with the amino acid tyrosine.

Tyrosine

Amino acids are the building blocks of protein, and this amino acid is a precursor to thyroid hormone. The body can make it from other amino acids, but meat, dairy and wheat are rich sources.

Other minerals required for thyroid function include calcium, chromium, magnesium, copper and iron. Essential vitamins include the B complex and vitamin C.

DIETARY FACTORS AFFECTING THYROID FUNCTION

Certain foods contain substances called *goitrogens*, which are believed to enlarge the thyroid and cause hypothyroidism by blocking the conversion of T4 hormone to T3. They can inhibit the body's ability to use iodine, which is essential for thyroid hormone synthesis. Foods which contain goitrogens include the brassica family: kale, sprouts, cauliflower, cabbage. Other goitrogenic foods include soya, radishes, watercress, mustard, turnips, cassava and peanuts.

As you can probably tell, these are, in fact, foods which we would ordinarily consider to be very healthy and desirable. A lot of people regularly eat green vegetables and other goitrogen-containing foods and they do not develop goitres or any other thyroid problem. There are two explanations for this: first, cooking these foods disables the goitrogens so they become harmless and, secondly, it is generally believed that eating moderate amounts of these foods is unlikely to have a negative effect on thyroid activity; it is thought that problems are only likely to arise where iodine is deficient.

Seaweed is an excellent, rich source of iodine. If you are vegetarian, vegan or avoid dairy and seafood, I would suggest adding edible seaweeds regularly to your diet. Once the preserve of the health food store, you can now buy these in most large supermarkets. Contrary to what you might think if you have never tried them before, they are in fact very tasty. They used to be a regular feature of the British diet, but sadly no more. Having said that, the current fashion for foraging in the wild might see seaweed make a much deserved comeback. It is rich in many minerals, not just iodine, and lends itself particularly well to stews and stir-fries. Nori, kombu, dulse and red seaweed (also called carragheen) are common staples. The Japanese make good use of seaweed in their traditional dishes and among the most popular are nori, wakame and arame – all of which are available in the UK.

Unless you know that you are iodine-deficient, it is not recommended that you start taking iodine supplements in the form of seaweed supplements, such as kelp, bladderwrack or bugleweed, because if you over-consume iodine you may put yourself at risk of developing hyperthyroidism. If in doubt, have yourself tested for iodine deficiency.

Case History

Michelle is a good case history because she was so typical, and because she illustrates how difficult it is to stimulate the thyroid through dietary measures alone. Michelle had plenty of symptoms of an underactive thyroid, but according to her GP's test results her thyroid was fine. Her main concern was her weight gain, and yes, she had a history of trying all sorts of rather bizarre diets. As a consequence she had put on about 2 stone and, despite her extraordinary self-discipline when it came to healthy eating and exercise, she just could not shift any weight. Not even a pound. She refused to go back to her doctor for more tests, and I was getting nowhere with her diet. Because her diet was so good and so varied (including plenty of dairy and seafood), and she also took a basic multivitamin and -mineral supplement, I felt it was unlikely that she was deficient in any of the nutrients essential for thyroid health. After a few visits I felt I had no option but to advise other therapies. So off Michelle went to a medical herbalist. The results were astonishing – in less than a month, she reported losing 2 lb. That might not sound much to you, but to Michelle it was extraordinary and uplifting. I lost touch with Michelle as she did not need to see me again, but the last time I heard from her she told me she had continued to lose more weight, albeit very slowly.

OTHER THERAPIES

As well as herbalism, I often recommend acupuncture as this therapy is particular useful for stimulating sluggish glands and organs. The thyroid can be incredibly stubborn but does often respond to the stimulating effects of acupuncture.

FURTHER INVESTIGATIONS

If you are highly stressed and suspect sub-clinical hypothyroidism, I would advise that you also read Solution 3: Overcoming Adrenal Fatigue. Stress is believed to inhibit thyroid function by decreasing production of TSH and inhibiting conversion of T4 to T3.[26] Therefore, by dealing with stress, you may find that your symptoms relating to mild underactive thyroid activity clear up.

Excessive oestrogen levels are known to suppress thyroid hormone, so if in addition to the symptoms of hypothyroidism you also experience symptoms associated with PMS or the menopause, I advise you to read Solution 5: Reversing Oestrogen Dominance.

Solution 7
Beating Gut Dysbiosis

Of all bodily functions, little surpasses the digestive process when it comes to causing embarrassment and repulsion. Funny noises, bad smells and even pain are for many people the penalty for one of our greatest pleasures, eating. Thus we may come to hate our own guts. They appear to conspire to torment and humiliate, shaming us for being human.

Those same guts which cause so much distress are really not your own. If you have ever thought that your innards appear to have a life of their own, it's because, in a sense, they have. Down there in that dark, murky area of your being exists a parallel universe of invisible microorganisms: microbes, transients, opportunists and freeloaders all merrily coexisting along the tube that runs from your mouth to your anus. There they live, breed, feed, ferment, evolve, do battle and eventually die or just move on out. So busy are these microorganisms that their combined metabolic activity has often been likened to that of the liver. You provide bacteria with a habitat; your body is their home but they are indifferent to you and your concerns. Even so, it is an advantageous arrangement: in exchange for food and shelter you get a great deal, as we shall see. Rather like small birds pecking insects off the backs of tolerant buffalo, bacteria clean up our digestive tract as part of a tacit, mutually agreeable arrangement we have with them.

An awful lot of bacteria are indigenous to the human body. There are approximately ten times as many bacteria in the human gut as there are cells in the body. There are around 400 to 500 species of 'normal' bacteria in the digestive system, and many strains of each type. Around 20 types of bacteria make up the majority. In total there are approximately 100 trillion bacteria in the gut, creating a weight of around 4 lb and contributing 40 to 60 per cent of the stool mass. Remember that the next time you peer down the lav to examine the denouement of your diet.

The presence of vast colonies of bacteria in the gut was discovered in the late 19th century. So repulsed were many sensitive (yet solvent) individuals by that discovery that they had their colons removed by the royal surgeon Sir William Arbuthnot Lane as treatment for what was termed 'intestinal toxaemia'. Today we have come to terms with the residents within, but to a large extent still fail to grasp their significance. When babies pick up all sorts of foul items and cram them into their tiny mouths, we recoil in horror before snatching away the offending object. This oral 'fixation' is firmly established as one of Sigmund Freud's stages of psychosexual development, where the infant derives immense gratification from oral stimulation. But I can't help wondering if Freud was totally *au fait* with the child's urgent need to colonize the gut with bacteria in order to build immunity as fast as possible. That is, of course, a rather more prosaic take on this reflex action but nonetheless one worthy of consideration.

DEFINING DYSBIOSIS

Just as humankind has managed to lay waste to the external ecology, so too do we frequently trash our own internal ecology. Dysbiosis is the opposite of symbiosis; it is dissonance instead of harmony. The term was first coined by Dr Elie Metchnikoff, who won the Nobel Prize in 1908 for his work on lactobacilli bacteria and their role in immunity. He used it to describe a state of imbalance of intestinal bacteria, or altered gut microflora. Dysbiosis is a state whereby an overgrowth of pathogenic, or 'bad' bacteria and other undesirable microorganisms creates harmful effects by changing their metabolic activity and colonizing the gut in greater than normal amounts. The activity of these dysfunctional bacteria, it is believed, results in the release of potentially toxic products which may play a role in many conditions.

Common symptoms associated with gut dysbiosis include:

- constipation

- diarrhoea/loose stools

- bloating

- excessive gas

- abdominal discomfort

- abdominal pain

- fatigue

- 'foggy' brain.

People normally come to see me with digestive problems because they have already consulted their GP and/or undergone various tests but haven't received a diagnosis because the tests proved negative. This suggests to me that the problem may be either dysbiosis or food sensitivity (see Solution 1 chapter). Gut dysbiosis normally occurs an hour or so after eating – clients often comment they feel fine on waking and that their symptoms only emerge after breakfast or lunch. Sometimes they say that symptoms developed immediately after a visit abroad, or after a course of antibiotics. These are all clues that point to dysbiosis, as we shall see further on. But first let's identify the good, the bad and the downright beastly, and the role they play in our health, or otherwise.

YOUR INVISIBLE FRIENDS (AND FOES)

There are two main groups of what are often referred to as 'friendly' bacteria in the gut: the lactic acid bacteria, and the bifidobacteria. The best known lactic acid bacteria are *L. acidophilus*, *L. bulgaricus* and *L. casei*. These bacteria are considered 'commensal' in that they are natural human gut inhabitants. The friendly bacteria are essential for human health: in exchange for our good health, we give them a nice warm, dark environment with lots of food to feed on.

The main pathogenic, or 'bad' bacteria are the bacteroides, plus shigella, klebsiella, entamoeba, streptococcus, clostridia and staphylococcus. The bacteroides are in fact normal inhabitants of the colon and form a large component of colonic bacteria. Even so, they are opportunistic pathogens frequently associated with gut infections and diarrhoea.

Until birth, the digestive tract is a sterile environment. The birth process puts paid to that, as bacteria are picked up along the birth canal, initiating the colonization process. The next source is touch and breastfeeding. Breastfeeding significantly influences the development of flora, as microbial life is known. Breastfed children quickly develop gut flora dominated by the lactic acid bacteria and bifidobacteria, especially *Bifido infantis*. Bottle-fed babies have much lower levels of bifidobacteria and their flora contains more bacteroides. As a result they have greater susceptibility to infection by pathogenic bacteria.

It is well known and accepted that breastfeeding is superior to bottle-feeding, and one of the reasons for this is the protective effect against infection conferred by breastfeeding. The gut flora of the breastfed infant has been shown to reduce the incidence of diarrhoea.[1] When weaning begins, the change to solid food marks the development of typical adult flora.

The adult digestive tract, which is effectively a muscular tube, measures about 11 metres from mouth to anus. The surface of the lining of the gut serves as a barrier which prevents a broad spectrum of undesirables from crossing over into the blood. At the same time this lining, which acts like an internal bouncer, has to be able to identify the desirables, specifically nutrients, and let them through.

The start of the digestive system is the mouth, where food is chewed and mixed with saliva secreted by salivary glands. This saliva softens up food and contains an enzyme called amylase which starts the process of digesting carbohydrates. When you swallow, food passes down the oesophagus, through the oesophageal sphincter and into the stomach.

The stomach has few bacteria, thanks to the presence of hydrochloric acid – few living organisms can withstand such an acidic environment, which is a good thing when you consider how easily all sorts of critters can find their way onto your plate. Fortunately, the stomach has a protective lining which prevents it being dissolved by its own acid. The stomach, which can hold about 1.5 litres of fluid, is like an industrial food-mixer. Food is mulched, kneaded and liquefied into a squelch called *chyme*. Protein digestion begins in the stomach via the action of hydrochloric acid and an enzyme called pepsin. Only water, some medicines and alcohol pass through the stomach wall, which explains that hit you get when drinking on an empty stomach.

After a couple of hours or so of this activity, liquefied food passes through the pyloric valve and enters the first part of the small intestine, the duodenum. The small intestine (which is about 7 metres long) is where food is digested and absorbed. It is lined with microscopic, finger-like protrusions called *villi* which in turn are covered with *microvilli*. These microvilli are an essential part of absorption.

In the first part of the duodenum, enzymes pour in from the pancreas. There are three types of enzymes: lipase (to digest fats), amylase (to digest carbohydrates) and protease (to digest protein). The pancreas also secretes bicarbonates in order to neutralize the acid from the stomach, and insulin to regulate blood-sugar levels. Bile from the liver emulsifies fats, making them more water-soluble so that enzymes can start digesting them.

The first part of the small intestine is colonized mainly by lactic acid bacteria, in particular *L. acidophilus.* There may also be small numbers of *E. coli* (the good kind, as opposed to the killer kind), yeast and a few other microorganisms. In the lower part of the small intestine the dominant group are the bifidobacteria, with some lactobacilli and streptococci. Food moves swiftly through the small intestine, and bacteria, in order to avoid being swept away, are able to adhere to the gut lining (the epithelium). However, many of these lactic acid bacteria are shed when food passes through, and the effect of this is to lower the pH of the gut, which has a protective effect against pathogens.

Further down, following digestion and absorption, food passes into the large intestine via the ileocaecal valve. The large intestine, also known as the colon, is around 3–5 feet long. Here, remaining nutrients and water are absorbed and some B vitamins are produced. The vast majority of bacteria in the gut are found in the colon. They are mainly bacteroides, though there are still significant numbers of bifidobacteria. After passing along the ascending, transverse and descending colon, the deconstructed food, now known as faeces, passes into the rectum. Here faeces are held until there is sufficient volume to create a bowel movement. A muscular wave, known as peristalsis, causes the faeces to pass out of the anus as stools. Stools are composed of undigested fibre, water, food metabolites and bacteria, both living and dead.

WHAT BACTERIA DO FOR US

The indigenous bacteria are often described as 'friendly', not because of their cheerful disposition but because of the work they do, albeit unwittingly, to promote our health. Human gut bacteria are essential to the health of the whole body, not just the digestive system. These bacteria perform a number of tasks, in particular those outlined below.

Kill Pathogens

Our microbial friends perform the extremely important task of controlling and preventing the overgrowth of unfriendly, even downright hostile bacteria which, if left to flourish, can cause unpleasant symptoms or disease. As well as inhibiting the overgrowth of 'bad' bacteria, such as salmonella, Escherichia coli (E. coli 0157) and H. pylori (the microbe now known to cause stomach ulcers), they also keep yeasts such as the various candida species in check. Obviously they do not do all this for purely altruistic reasons: by blocking their competitors they are able to flourish and survive more easily. They do this in a number of ways:

They Create an Acid Environment

Lactobacillus bacteria such as *L. acidophilus* feed on carbohydrates, and produce lactic acid in the process. This lactic acid lowers the pH of the gut to around 4.0, and this inhibits most other microbes. *E. coli* 0157, for example, is a disease-causing microbe which is inactivated in an environment with a pH below 5. The lactic acid bacteria also produce hydrogen peroxide, which inhibits the growth of yeasts such as *Candida albicans*.

They Produce Natural Antibiotic Factors

Friendly bacteria, especially *L. acidophilus*, are able to manufacture antibiotic substances, namely lactocidin, lactobacillin, lactobreven and acidolin. These can inhibit pathogenic bacteria, including salmonella and *E. coli*. The bifidobacteria, on the other hand, are effective against pathogenic bacteria in a different way: they produce bacteriocins, proteins which are antagonistic to bacteria such as listeria and enterococcus.

They Produce Short-chain Fatty Acids

The bifidobacteria, which inhabit mainly the colon, produce short-chain fatty acids (SCFAs), the most abundant being acetic acid. Acetic acid exerts powerful activity against yeasts and bad bacteria.

They Create Spatial Exclusion

In sufficient quantities, they constitute an 'army' which crowds out invading pathogens along the intestinal lining, preventing bad bacteria, parasites and so on from getting a look-in.

Build Immunity

Gut flora stimulates and influences the immune system, and disturbances in the population of the gut can damage immunity. In animals devoid of intestinal bacteria, i.e. which have been bred to have a sterile gut, severe infections occur with little chance of survival.[2] Both lactobacilli and bifidobacteria strengthen the ability of immune cells in the gut lining to defend against toxins and pathogenic microorganisms, as well as allergens (substances which trigger an allergic response). They do this through:

- **Stimulation of the production of antibodies.** With the assistance of good bacteria, the gut makes secretory immunoglobulin A (SigA), an antibody which binds to pathogens, preventing them from attaching themselves to the gut lining.

- **Stimulation of gut-associated lymphoid tissue (GALT).** GALT represents approximately 60 per cent of the human immune system. Indeed, this GALT constitutes the largest lymphoid organ in the body, and it is highly sensitive to fluctuations in bacterial activity.

- **Prevention of inflammation.** Some bacteria can actually improve the symptoms of inflammatory bowel disorder (IBD) through their anti-inflammatory activity.

Improve Digestion

Friendly bacteria encourage peristalsis and therefore motility of food through the gut, helping to prevent constipation and keeping the bowels regular. Lactic acid bacteria such as *L. acidophilus* produce the enzyme lactase, which is necessary for the digestion of milk sugar (lactose). They also help digest proteins and break down bile acids. As we saw in the Solution 5 chapter, bacteria metabolize plant compounds which are then absorbed into the blood and help normalize oestrogen levels.

Provide Energy

Bacteroides in the colon produce enzymes that ferment and digest dietary fibre, and this fermentation produces short-chain fatty acids – butyrate, propionate, acetate and valerate – which are then absorbed into the blood. Acetate and propionate provide energy for the brain, muscle and the heart, while butyrate provides about half of the daily energy requirements of the gut lining.

Protect Against Heart Disease and Cancer

The short-chain fatty acids produced by the fermentation of fibre are protective against heart disease and cancer.[3] One way they do this is by helping to regulate cholesterol and circulating fat levels. Chronic heart failure is due in part to inflammation, and it has been found that disturbed gut bacteria can trigger the inflammation which leads to this condition.[4]

We have seen that the short-chain fatty acids, produced by the fermentation of carbohydrates by bacteria, provide the body with energy. One of those SCFAs, butyrate, is directly involved in cancer prevention. Butyrate has been shown to kill cancer cells and stimulate the growth of normal cells.[5] Friendly bacteria can also prevent the growth of those bacteria that produce nitrates in the colon, which are known to cause cancer of the bowel.

Remove Inorganic Toxins

Along with food, we ingest all manner of non-food substances, some of which are natural, some of which are very unnatural. Friendly bacteria help us break down and eliminate toxic substances such as drugs, food additives, mercury, pesticides and other pollutants.

Produce Vitamins and Promote the Absorption of Minerals

Lactic acid bacteria manufacture, through their metabolic processes, vitamins B_1, B_2, B_3, B_5, B_6, B_{12}, folate, biotin and vitamin K. Lactic acid bacteria promote the absorption of minerals which require acid for absorption – iron, calcium, magnesium and copper.

THE EFFECTS OF DYSBIOSIS

Dysbiosis has been indicated in numerous health crimes because the products of bacterial metabolism are distributed systemically in the bloodstream. As well as reducing your overall immunity and increasing your risk of cancer and heart disease, dysbiosis is also linked to conditions affecting the nervous system, including chronic fatigue syndrome. As far as digestive health is concerned, there are two main areas where dysbiosis really does its worst: it contributes to inflammatory bowel disease and encourages the proliferation of pathogenic microorganisms – parasites, yeasts and other hangers-on – which are then free to vandalize with impunity.

Inflammatory Bowel Disease (IBD)

IBD is a general term used to describe a group of chronic inflammatory disorders affecting the bowel, of which the two main types are Crohn's disease and ulcerative colitis.

Crohn's mainly affects the colon but may in fact involve any part of the digestive system. The affected area is thickened with ulceration and the formation of fistulas. The main symptoms are pain, diarrhoea and weight loss. As a result of the damage to the intestinal wall, malabsorption occurs. Overgrowth of pathogenic bacteria has been found in studies of patients with this disease, though the only microorganism reported to be strongly associated with Crohn's disease is *E. coli*.[6]

Ulcerative colitis is a chronic inflammatory condition of the large bowel and is characterized by bloody diarrhoea. Mucus is also passed in the stool. There are usually cramps in the lower abdomen, with mild abdominal tenderness.

Dysbiosis is very much linked to IBD, and the bacteroides and other unfriendly bacteria are found to be increased in people with IBD, with significantly reduced numbers of bifidobacteria.[7] Studies have repeatedly found different bacterial activity between people with IBD and healthy controls. It is believed that dysbiosis may disturb the partnership between flora and the human immune system, and the effect this has on the immune system may create responses that underlie inflammatory disorders.[8]

Overgrowth of Pathogenic Microorganisms

Bacteria

Dysbiosis can create increased vulnerability to pathogenic bacteria such as salmonella, shigella and klebsiella. Salmonella is probably the best known, and causes severe gastrointestinal illness accompanied by pain, cramping, nausea and vomiting. The condition usually resolves without treatment. Shigella causes dysentery. In the UK the effect of shigella infection is usually mild, with some abdominal pain and diarrhoea. It can also cause 'traveller's diarrhoea' and in some people symptoms can be severe. *Klebsiella pneumoniae* is the most common form of klebsiella in hospital patients and can cause pneumonia in susceptible individuals. The most common cause of food poisoning in Britain is the bacterium campylobacter, which is found in raw meat.

Parasites

Parasites may be intestinal or blood-borne. In the intestines they are either single-celled microorganisms or helminths – worms, such as roundworm or tapeworm. Worms are generally visible to the naked eye, but not so your single-celled parasites. These include various types of amoeba (the most common types are *Endolimax nana*, *Dientamoeba fragilis*, *Entamoeba histolytica*), giardia (most commonly *G. lamblia*), *Blastocystis hominis* and cryptosporidium. They may cause no symptoms at all, but if there is an overgrowth, or you are elderly or have a compromised immune system, there are a number of symptoms you may experience if you have one or more of these parasites: abdominal pain, diarrhoea (sometimes alternating with constipation), flatulence, bloating, lower back pain, weight loss and fatigue.

When I mention the possibility of parasites to clients, a shadow of horror usually passes over their faces. That is because we tend to think of parasites as hairy, bug-eyed beasts trawling through our guts, rather than as invisible microorganisms. They are extraordinarily common, yet rarely considered by medics. When I talk to my clients who have been trying to deal with their digestive problems for years, and have trolled back and forth to their GP for the duration, I find that any discussion of parasites has rarely occurred. How common is parasitic infection? There doesn't appear to be any data for the UK, but US studies are interesting. In 1987 a survey by the Centers for Disease Control showed a frequency of positivity in 2.6 per cent of laboratory samples. By 2000, however, a third of stool samples from 2,896 patients in the US tested positive for intestinal parasites, and, of those, 23 per cent were infected with *Blastocystis hominis*.[9] Globalization of our lifestyles has led to globalization of our diseases, so it is no wonder that *B. hominis* and others easily make their way round the world.

If I suspect a client may have intestinal parasites there are certain questions I always ask. These include: Have you done much travelling recently? Did your symptoms come on suddenly? Do you get painful cramps in the abdomen area? Do you get frequent diarrhoea? A positive answer to any of these questions raises my suspicions, and at this point I often suggest a lab test. If the test result is positive, the culprit is almost always, in my experience, *B. hominis*. The symptoms commonly associated with *Blastocystis* – which is able to lodge in the intestinal wall, making it hard to eradicate – are abdominal pain, bloating, cramps, occasional diarrhoea, constipation, aching joints and skin rash. Mental symptoms include fatigue, lassitude and dizziness. Transmission is believed to be faecal/oral – a nice way of saying poor toilet hygiene on the part of whoever has cooked or served the offending food. Other parasites are water-borne – giardia and cryptosporidium are resistant to chlorine and can spread through drinking water.

Yeast Overgrowth

There are all sorts of yeasts co-habiting in your gut, and if you have a healthy gut flora they do no harm. However, this balance can go awry if your friendly bacteria are insufficient in number to keep them under control, or if you have poor gut immunity or inadequate intestinal pH levels.

The most commonly found yeasts include *Candida krusei*, *Candida tropicalis* and *Geotrichum*. However, most common of all is *Candida albicans*. Ordinarily, *C. albicans* thrives in an alkaline environment, so is controlled by lactic acid bacteria. The hydrogen peroxide also produced by *L. acidophilus* kills candida directly. Given the right circumstances, candida, like all yeasts, can flourish and proliferate, and any unchecked growth of their colonies can be explosive, resulting in the production of powerful toxins. Yeasts particularly like warm dark places, so the gastrointestinal tract and vagina, where it manifests as thrush, are particularly accommodating.

It is believed that *C. albicans* is able to break down the digestive system's front line of defence against infectious agents, the antibody SigA.[10] The most common physical symptoms of *C. albicans* overgrowth are abdominal discomfort, constipation and/or diarrhoea, PMS and recurring urinary tract infections, sore muscles and acne. There may also be fungal infection in the nails, eyes and on the skin, as well as vaginal thrush. The most common mental symptoms include depression, fuzzy thinking, poor memory and concentration, insomnia, mood swings and fatigue. Sensitivity to perfumes, detergents and other chemicals is not uncommon.

Unlike many other organisms, candida does nothing useful for us and is a true parasite. It can colonize the entire digestive tract, from mouth to anus. In the mouth it is visible as white spots and a coated tongue. It can cause itching around the anus and discharge of mucus. No wonder, then, that people who genuinely have a yeast overgrowth tend to feel sick all over, as if the whole body feels toxic.

The reason for candida's systemic assault lies in its ability to change from a yeast form to a fungal form. When it does so, it develops rhizoids, which are rather like the roots of a plant. These roots are able to penetrate the gut lining and enter the bloodstream. Candida is then free to travel the body, wreaking havoc as it does so. So too are other toxic substances, thanks to the gut permeability created by the rhizoids. For more about this see Solution 8, which is about leaky gut syndrome.

GETTING TO THE BOTTOM OF IT

If you have any number of digestive symptoms, you need to find out what exactly is causing them in order to get the appropriate treatment. This means going to your GP and, if necessary, undergoing one or more tests. Your GP might suggest testing for *Helicobacter pylori*, the bacterium now known to cause stomach ulcers. A breath test is a common procedure for this. Tests will also help eliminate any concerns about bowel cancer, the third most common cancer and the second most common cause of cancer death in the UK. Tests frequently undertaken include sigmoidoscopy, colonoscopy or endoscopy. A colonoscopy is an examination of the rectum for abnormalities, including tumour. A sigmoidoscopy is similar, and looks at the lining of the colon and may involve taking a biopsy. An endoscopy involves inserting a camera probe into the stomach and the duodenum to investigate the presence of an ulcer or tumour.

Another means of examining the bowel for growths is a barium enema, a type of X-ray which involves inserting a tube into the rectum. The inside of the bowel is first coated with a powder called barium sulphate to produce a clearer image. A barium enema is used to examine the large bowel (colon and rectum) for problems such as growths (polyps), inflammation (colitis), and tumours. Barium sulphate can also be given as a drink (barium meal) to examine the upper intestinal tract (endoscopy).

If tests reveal nothing untoward, your GP may diagnose you with irritable bowel syndrome.

IRRITABLE BOWEL SYNDROME

This is a popular diagnosis where there are plenty of symptoms but no known cause. According to The Gut Trust – 'the national charity for IBS' – between 10 and 20 per cent of people living in Western countries fulfil the diagnostic criteria for IBS alone – and this figure does not even include other disorders of the gut. A diagnosis is made where there is abdominal pain and altered bowel habit. This pain may be in any area of the abdomen, but most frequently in the lower left or right hand side. There may be either constipation or diarrhoea, or alternate episodes of both. There may also be bloating, excessive gas and a feeling of incomplete emptying after a bowel movement. There is no specific remedy.

I may be a cynic, but I have a theory concerning IBS. I see it as an umbrella term, which, when offered as a diagnosis, could be taken to mean: there is something wrong with your digestive system but we don't know what. Neither do we know what to do about it. Try these antispasmodic drugs. Then again, you may be imagining it all. Try these antidepressants.

It is generally agreed by specialists in the area that the treatment for IBS is neither evidence-based, nor efficient.[11] That is probably why management often means advising patients that they have to come to terms with their symptoms, perhaps with the help of some antidepressants. I have seen many people who have been totally disillusioned by the lack of effective advice given and who consequently refused the treatment offered. I strongly suspect that IBS and dysbiosis are one and the same thing, especially as studies have shown that probiotics (friendly bacteria in supplement form) are equally effective as antispasmodic drugs in the alleviation of IBS symptoms.[12] In the US, a parasitic infection is found in almost half of diagnosed cases of IBS where testing has occurred. Indeed, the symptoms of IBS and *B. hominis* infection have been shown to be 'remarkably similar'. Some researchers even believe that IBS may be caused by *B. hominis*.[13] The problem in the UK is that, because no one usually looks for parasitic infection, it is not usually found.

WHAT CAUSES DYSBIOSIS?

Under certain circumstances the microflora of the gut can be altered, and indeed severely disrupted. The main, non-diet related issues are discussed below. Diet-related causes of dysbiosis are discussed in the 'Return to Balance' section (page 154).

Drugs

Certain drugs, including steroids and the contraceptive pill, are known to disturb the human gut microflora, but no drug can obliterate gut bacteria quite the way that antibiotics can.

Antibiotics are not discriminatory; instead they annihilate the good with the bad. *Lactobacillus aciphophilus* can be virtually wiped out by a course of antibiotics. This clears a path for hostile bacteria, parasites and pathogenic yeasts to thrive. These include *E. coli*, staphylococci, streptococci and yeasts, notably *Candida albicans* – yeasts are especially free to proliferate, as they are not affected by antibiotics.

Even if you don't take antibiotics you will ingest them in the meats you eat because antibiotics are routinely used in livestock, not just to treat disease but as a preventative measure in intensive farming – cramming animals together in closed buildings makes them vulnerable to infection. As a result, meat contains antibiotic residues, as do milk and milk products.

Stress

There is plenty of evidence to demonstrate that stress has a significant influence over the activity of bacteria in the gut, however strange this may seem. You might think those tiny blighters would be indifferent to your feelings, but you'd be wrong. They too are sensitive, but in a more opportunistic than solicitous manner.

We saw in the Solution 3 chapter how stress can cause a dramatic rise in adrenal cortisol levels, cortisol being a major stress hormone. When a group of stressed-out students had saliva and faecal samples taken during the start of a semester and also during the first week of exams (in other words, during periods of low and high stress) researchers found significantly lower levels of lactic acid bacteria during the high-stress condition, when cortisol levels were found to be high.[14] This suggests that stress can actually be involved in the initiation of infectious disease, as well as non-infectious diseases such as heart disease and cancer, because of the way it changes the activity of the gut flora. The immune system and the central nervous system are known to 'cross-talk', and perception of stress by the nervous system causes the release of stress hormones. Infectious, pathogenic bacteria have evolved detection systems to sense stress hormones and then use them to proliferate and initiate infection.[15] What cunning little deviants those pathogens truly are.

Age

The elderly are prone to dysbiosis because they have an altered microflora, with decreased numbers of beneficial bacteria. People aged over 55 have been shown to have a marked decrease in levels of bifidobacteria, which may make them more susceptible to infection.[16] This decrease in numbers is possibly due to reduced ability of the bacteria to adhere to the gut lining.[17] With fewer friendly bacteria, intestinal immunity is compromised and this can lead to *Clostridium difficile*-related diarrhoea, one of the most common gastrointestinal infections in the elderly. Antibiotics, not surprisingly, exacerbate dysbiosis in the elderly.[18] It is not difficult to imagine the domino-like consequences of frequent antibiotic therapy in the elderly.

RETURN TO BALANCE

There are foods which encourage the proliferation of friendly bacteria, and other foods and food components which have the opposite effect, stimulating yeasts and pathogenic organisms so that they flourish. Hence you need to know which foods to avoid and which ones to consume in copious quantities in order to create bacterial harmony in your gut.

Fibre

You know fibre is good for you. All that roughage sweeps debris through your colon and keeps you regular. It does lots of good things, like removing cholesterol, old hormones and a variety of toxins, carcinogens and waste from the body. Fibre also provides sustenance for your friendly fauna, and a low-fibre diet encourages the proliferation of bad bacteria.

Fibre is usually categorized as being either soluble or insoluble. High-fibre foods tend to contain a mix of both types. The insoluble type is particularly good because it favours the proliferation of friendly bacteria.

Insoluble Fibre

Insoluble fibre forms part of the plant cell wall, giving structure to plants. It is indigestible so passes unabsorbed through the body, taking toxins, carcinogens and other waste products with it. Insoluble fibre helps prevent constipation by keeping matter moving along, speeding up transit time, absorbing water and making stools soft and therefore comfortable to pass. This non-digestible fibre also appears able to exert beneficial influences on the composition and activity of gut bacteria.[19] Undigested fibre is fermented by bacteria in the colon, and this fermentation produces gases (carbon dioxide, hydrogen and methane) and short-chain fatty acids, as described above (page 142).

Good sources of insoluble fibre include:

* fruits

* vegetables, especially celery and sweetcorn

* beans and lentils

* oats

* wholegrains, such as brown rice and wheat.

Soluble Fibre

Soluble fibre can be partially digested; its beneficial properties include its ability to reduce blood cholesterol and blood pressure, help control blood-sugar levels and reduce the risk of certain diseases such as diabetes and gallstones.

Good sources of soluble fibre include:

- oats

- beans and lentils

- fruits – especially berries, apples, pears and citrus fruits

- vegetables

- barley.

Some fibres are partially soluble, such as the oligosaccharides. An oligosaccharide is a short chain of sugar molecules (*oligo* means 'few' and *saccharide* means 'sugar'). Fructo-oligosaccharides are a type of oligosaccharide composed of fructose (fruit sugar) molecules and are found in bananas and other fruits, Jerusalem artichokes, onions, barley, garlic, wheat, asparagus, burdock, leeks and chicory. Oligosaccharides are only partially digested, and it is the undigested portion which serves as food for friendly bacteria and stimulates their growth. They have other properties, too: some are potent inhibitors of bacterial adhesion – that is, they stop bad bacteria from sticking to the gut lining. This action helps protect against infectious agents, including *E. coli*.[20] Oligosaccharides can significantly change the composition of gut bacteria by favouring the proliferation of friendly bacteria without favouring the bad bacteria.[21]

Sugar and Refined Carbohydrates

Nothing is as tasty to pathogenic yeasts and other undesirable microorganisms as sugar, sugary foods and refined carbohydrates, devoid of helpful fibre. These pathogens have to eat too, and these are their preferred foods.

Consumption of refined sugar has been implicated in many gut disorders and is associated with the development of colon cancer, gallstones and Crohn's disease.[22] A high-sugar diet has also been found to slow down transit time and significantly alter bacterial activity.[23] Slow transit time means that undesirable bacteria have more time to flourish and more fodder on which to dine.

The effect of sugar on microorganisms can be observed right at the beginning of the digestive tract. Sugars, including glucose and sucrose (but not the milk sugar lactose) have been found to significantly promote the adhesion of pathogenic yeasts, namely candida, to the cells of the mouth.[24] Sugary foods and refined carbohydrates should be totally excluded from the diet of anyone with gut dysbiosis. This includes fruit juices but not fruit itself, which is a fantastic source of fibre as well as nutrients which help feed the friendly bacteria.

Fermented Foods

The tradition of fermenting foods is ancient in certain parts of the world, especially Asia, Africa and Eastern Europe. Bacteria, or a mixture of bacteria and yeasts, can be employed in the fermentation process; the result is increased good bacteria content. Fermenting foods also extends their shelf life. Probably the best-known fermented food is live, or 'bio' yoghurt. Another well-known fermented product is kefir, a fermented milk drink thought to originate centuries ago in the Caucasus mountains. Other fermented foods include sauerkraut, cottage cheese and certain soya bean products: tofu, miso, tempeh, tamari and shoyu.

Tamari and shoyu are types of soya sauce. Tempeh is soya bean paste fermented with a mould called *Rhizopus oligosporous* and used as a meat substitute. It has a chewy texture and can be fried, baked or steamed. Soya beans can be fermented with rice and barley to make a condiment called miso, using a fungus called *Aspergillus oryzae*. Miso is usually added to soups, sauces and stews. Tofu is soya bean curd. The beans are soaked and crushed and then heated to produce soya milk, which is then coagulated to form a curd. It can be added to curries and stews as a meat substitute, though it is rather bland. It does helpfully soak up other flavours, which makes it more palatable. Like meat and fish, it is a complete protein – so ideal for vegetarians and vegans.

Cruciferous Vegetables

As you may have noticed by now, these vegetables are true multi-taskers, keeping blood sugar regular, fighting cancer and balancing hormones. Another feather in the cruciferous cap is their ability to favour your friendly bacteria. Vegetables such as cauliflower, broccoli, sprouts and cabbage contain compounds called glucosinolates which can be fermented and used as fuel by bacteria, making them *prebiotics* – foods which feed benign bacteria. You couldn't design a more human-friendly vegetable. Along with glucosinolates, they also contain something called sulforaphane, which in experiments has been shown to inhibit the growth of the bacterial pathogen *Helicobacter pylori*, which causes stomach ulcers. Indeed, it has been found that sulforaphane inhibits 23 out of 28 different types of disease-causing bacteria.[25] So a sprout isn't just for Christmas – it's for as many days of the year as you can manage.

Fat and Protein

Interestingly, fat has been shown to have no effect on bacterial activity, with the exception of fish oil, which in animal studies has been shown to decrease the bacteroides and increase the good bifidobacteria.[26] Unfortunately there have been very few studies on the effects of fat and protein on microbial activity, though one useful study compared the diets of strict vegetarians with people eating a general 'Western' diet and found no difference in the types of gut bacteria found in both groups, leading the researchers to conclude that dietary intake of animal fat and protein does not appear to alter gut bacteria.[27] Having said that, how well you actually digest the protein you eat does appear to make a big difference. It is especially important that food is properly digested, especially protein, by the time it reaches the colon. The best way to ensure adequate digestion is to chew food thoroughly so that your digestive enzymes can get at it and do their job efficiently. Undigested proteins may start to ferment and this creates harmful substances such as ammonia and amines, which are associated with the growth of potentially pathogenic bacteria.[28] Ammonia is thought to be especially toxic to the gut lining.

PROBIOTICS, PREBIOTICS AND ANTI-FUNGALS

Probiotics are foods and supplements containing live bacteria, and prebiotics are foods and supplements containing foods which feed and encourage friendly bacteria to proliferate. Supplemental probiotics are usually sourced from the bifidobacteria or lactobacilli groups and are of human origin.

It was the aforementioned Dr Elie Metchnikoff who introduced the concept of probiotics at the beginning of the 20th century and who described the good health and longevity of Bulgarian peasants who consumed large quantities of fermented milk. How Sir William Arbuthnot Lane, he of the famous colon-removal approach to digestive health, explained this development to his colon-less clients is not documented, as far as I am aware, even though these two eminent gentlemen were contemporaries.

Probiotics and prebiotics are currently among the most researched natural products, because they are proving to be of enormous benefit to human health. Indeed, use of probiotics and prebiotics is believed to play a role in the prevention and treatment of a number of diseases, including inflammatory bowel disorders, arthritis, allergy and colon cancer.[29] There is substantial evidence to show that probiotics and prebiotics can protect against the production of toxins in the gut.[30] Perhaps their best feature is their ability to control inflammation. Probiotics do this not only in the gut, but also, via their metabolic end-products, throughout the body. In the gut itself, supplemental probiotics have been found to be effective in preventing and treating antibiotic-associated diarrhoea, and in suppressing overgrowth of candida which can arise as a consequence of antibiotic therapy.[31] Supplemental prebiotics have been found to increase bifidobacteria and lactobacillus whilst decreasing bacteroides and candida.[32] Other reported benefits of prebiotics include an improvement in the absorption of minerals in the large bowel.[33]

We have seen how the ageing process results in a reduction in levels of friendly bacteria in the gut. Many now agree that supplementing probiotics may be beneficial for the elderly, as research suggests that probiotics may improve their immune system.[34] Specifically, giving elderly people supplements of *Bifidobacterium lactis* has been shown to increase levels of T-lymphocytes and natural killer cells, important components of the immune system[35] For this reason it is thought that giving supplements to the elderly in care who have received broad-spectrum antibiotic treatment may be of benefit.[36]

Survival of the Fittest

The main challenge associated with supplemental bacteria lies in their ability to survive the hostile, highly acidic environment of the stomach so that they arrive at their final destination, the intestines. Studies have shown that not all commercial products are equal to this challenge. To have any therapeutic effect, very large numbers of probiotic bacteria are required.[37] No one actually knows precisely what figure we should be aiming for, but it can be assumed that, given the low pH of the stomach and the harsh environment of the digestive tract, more really is more. Most nutritional therapists would not consider a supplement that contained less than one billion viable cells, and usually look for a probiotic/prebiotic combination. Combining probiotics with prebiotics in supplement form can promote and enhance the survival of the former.[38]

Anti-fungal Agents

There is a substantial number of plant and plant extracts which have been shown to have anti-fungal activity, and these can be taken in the diet, in supplement form or as a tea or drink. Anti-fungals commonly used by nutritional therapists include:

- caprylic acid from coconut

- garlic

- oleic acid from olive oil

- pau d'arco (available as a tea)

- grapefruit seed extract

- biotin (a B vitamin)

- aloe vera juice

- oregano oil

- berberine-containing plants (*Berberis vulgaris, Berberis aquifolium*).

Some of these substances also have anti-parasitic effects, especially berberine, garlic, grapefruit seed extract and oregano. Other anti-parasitic agents include black walnut and wormwood.

TESTING

How do you know whether or not you have dysbiosis, and if so whether or not you additionally harbour a yeast overgrowth or even a parasitic infection? How do you tell the difference? This is a particularly tricky question, as symptoms are mainly non-specific. Perhaps you'd rather not know, which is fine because the diet you need to follow is the same regardless of what form of dysbiosis your guts have succumbed to. Some people just like to know their nemesis (lots of people, I find). If you are one of those people, there is only one way: a home stool test.

Before you gag, rest assured that this does not involve tipping a turd into a jiffy bag and then slipping out under cover of darkness to post it. It's much more dignified and hygienic, I'm happy to confirm.

Before I explain, let me first say that unfortunately the best, most accurate tests are simply not available on the NHS. NHS tests are not sensitive enough to detect microorganisms such as *Blastocystis hominis*, nor to examine the ratio of friendly to unfriendly bacteria. If you really want to know quite specifically what sort of microflora you possess, or whether or not you have parasites or a yeast infection, I recommend a comprehensive parasitology stool analysis.

This is a gem of a test as it takes all the guesswork out of identifying intestinal offenders. The comprehensive parasitology detects all the usual suspects, as well as some of the lesser spotted microbes, including *Blastocystis hominis* (without doubt the most frequently observed faecal parasite), cryptosporidium, various amoebae, flagellates and just about anything that has no right to be living off your metabolic processes.

The test involves three test tubes containing a formaldehyde solution. All you do is take a very small stool extract with the little spade provided, put it in the test tube, screw the top on and give it a good shake. Then you put the test tubes in the prepaid, pre-labelled bag marked 'my stool sample' (only kidding; it says no such thing) and put it in the post. For details of the comprehensive parasitology test see the Resources chapter.

WHAT SHOULD YOU DO?

Here is a step-by-step guide to reversing dysbiosis and its attendant overgrowths of pathogenic microorganisms.

* See your GP. You need to eliminate the possibility that you have an inflammatory bowel disorder, cancer or any other serious gastrointestinal disorder. Your GP may decide to run tests such as those described above. He or she may even decide to test you for giardiasis, one of the few parasitic infections for which NHS testing is available.

- If no medical diagnosis is forthcoming, you might want to consider the possibility that you have dysbiosis. If you feel you would like to test for this, see the Resources chapter. However, bear in mind that if you do indeed have dysbiosis, coupled with a parasitic infection, you should not attempt to tackle this without professional help. From the list of anti-parasitic agents (page 162) you can see that there are many plant extracts which can be deployed. Some of these are very powerful and you need to know what you are doing to get the correct dosage with the desired effect without side effects. I advise you to consult either a nutritional therapist experienced in dealing with parasites or a medical herbalist with similar experience. See the Resources chapter.

- If testing reveals you have a yeast overgrowth, such as *Candida albicans*, follow the diet advice below. I have seen many clients who, upon testing, find they do indeed have a yeast infection. However, a surprising number of people merely have dysbiosis without yeast overgrowth. *Candida albicans* overgrowth has been the diagnosis of far too many complementary therapists when dealing with just about any symptom, ranging from depression to diarrhoea. The traditional 'anti-candida' diet, so readily prescribed by so many complementary therapists, is severely restrictive and involves not only eliminating all refined carbohydrates and sugar, which is fair enough, but also fruit (because it contains fruit sugar so must be bad), mushrooms (because surely mushroom equals fungus equals bad) and fermented foods (because fermentation must be bad, too, as it suggests bacterial and yeast activity). Bread, tinned foods and many others are also prohibited. Despite there being no evidence to support this hairshirt regime, people frequently do embark upon it and end up feeling wretched when they fail to persevere for the prescribed number of weeks or months.

A few years ago I saw a client who came to me with what she believed to be recurrent thrush. She had been on the anti-candida diet for two years, on the advice of her reflexologist. To her credit, and my amazement, she had followed it strictly for that time, but she was miserable. In tears she told me she couldn't stand it any longer, especially as she still had thrush anyway. I thought it highly unlikely that any yeast, after two years of starvation, would have any hope of survival in any part of her body and advised that she see her GP for a test for something else – vaginosis. She did, and tested positive for *Gardnerella vaginalis*, not candida. Gardnerella, a bacterium, is a prime cause of vaginosis, a condition which causes symptoms similar to thrush but is not the same thing. Untreated, vaginosis can lead to complications in pregnancy and may increase your risk of developing pelvic inflammatory disease.

I must confess that in my early, evangelical days I too preached the doctrine of forbidden fruits (and the rest) with regard to *Candida albicans*, until I realized the non-necessity and impossibility of such a restrictive, punishing approach. Now I find that by making more moderate dietary alterations, pathogenic yeasts and other undesirable microorganisms retreat into harmlessness. Only occasionally is it necessary to resort to powerful anti-fungals. So if your test results suggest yeast overgrowth, or you suspect as much, consider the following dietary advice first. After a couple of weeks introduce probiotics (supplemented with prebiotics). You could also add gentle anti-fungals such as aloe vera juice and pau d'arco tea, both available from any health food shop. If this fails it is time to call in the professionals – but I suspect that in many cases this won't be necessary.

- If testing indicates dysbiosis without candida or parasites, simply follow the advice below. If you do not undergo testing but suspect dysbiosis, this programme should also prove to be well worth a try.

Diet for Dysbiosis

Eat lots of
Garlic, raw wherever possible
Olive oil – on everything
Vegetables – as many and as varied as possible
Cruciferous vegetables: sprouts, cabbage, kale, broccoli, cauliflower
Fruit – all that FOS
FOS-rich vegetables
All beans and lentils
Oats
Nuts and seeds
Live natural yoghurt
Tofu, tempeh and other fermented foods
Fish, especially oily fish
Avoid
Sugar
Anything with sugar added
Anything refined: white rice, pasta, pastry, etc.
Savoury snacks such as crisps, biscuits, etc.
High-glycaemic index foods (see Solution 2 chapter)

Restrict or avoid
Alcohol
Avoid beer completely
Neutral foods
Meat (buy organic to avoid those antibiotics)
Dairy (again, organic is better)
Eggs
White fish, shellfish

As you can see, this regime is not really too onerous. The 'eat lots of' column is pretty generous compared to the others. If you are making massive dietary changes, expect those to be reflected in your wind-breaking habits. Initially, expect to be unsociable as your gut adjusts to the changes in microbial activity. Once you adjust to all this fibre and goodness, so too will your overexcited friendly bacteria, and the windiness will calm down.

GERM THEORIES

Most people are now aware of the perils of indiscriminate antibiotic use. Antibiotics carpet-bomb the gut, destroying good and bad bacteria alike and with no preference for either. It is not difficult to imagine the consequences to your health of destroying those bacteria which are not just 'friendly' but which are an essential component of immunity against disease.

Antibiotics provide an opportunity for bacteria to mutate into bigger, stronger versions of themselves, requiring bigger, stronger antibiotics to wipe them out. This procedure has given rise to the aptly termed 'superbug' – antibiotic-resistant bacteria such as

MRSA. Bugs such as MRSA (methicillin-resistant *S. aureus*) didn't just arise naturally, or by chance: we bred them.

We've got ourselves into a right mess now. In order to contain the spread of superbugs, we have to use antibacterial sprays, wipes and other paraphernalia, which can only lead to further mutations of these bacteria, thereby reducing our resistance to ... antibiotic-resistant superbugs such as MRSA. Superbugs lead to superinfections. More scrupulous hygiene in hospitals has led to a decline in the incidence of MRSA infection, but other bacteria are flourishing, having outwitted their antibiotic nemeses. Shigella is showing increasing resistance, as is *Streptococcus pneumoniae*, enterococcus, klebsiella, *Citrobacter freundii*, *M. tuberculosis*, salmonella and *Helicobacter pylori*.[39] According to the UK Health Protection Agency, antibiotic use is a major contributor to the development of gastrointestinal disease, with the bacterium *Clostridium difficile* now commonly contracted in hospitals. Bacterial infections can spread like wildfire: with globalization of our lifestyles has come globalization of disease.

Another major factor in the creation of superbugs is the overuse of antibiotics on intensively reared livestock – farming has been implicated in the rise of both MRSA and *E. coli*.[40] The total volume of antibiotics used in the UK for farming purposes, in 2007, was 387 tonnes.[41] According to the Government's Chief Medical Officer, every time an antibiotic is used it becomes less effective in the population as a whole, and every unnecessary use of antibiotics in animals or agriculture 'is potentially signing a death warrant for a future patient'.[42]

It may be essential to use antibacterial products in hospitals and other environments where there are vulnerable and sick people at risk of infection, but what I find disturbing is the creeping insinuation from advertising that danger from germs lurks everywhere in our homes. Healthy people living in healthy environments do not need to sterilize every inch of their homes, despite cynical suggestions to the contrary.

The fact is it is futile to regard all bacteria as the enemy. There are some extremely dangerous, life-threatening bugs out there, and that is when antibiotics really come into their own. Certain conditions such as meningitis, pneumonia and septicaemia can be deadly without them. We can win certain battles, but the war is unwinnable: bacteria were here long before we were, and will still be here long after we are gone. Indeed, they are our oldest ancestors, the first form of life that appeared about 4 billion years ago. They still rule the Earth. They are present everywhere on the planet and in the Earth's crust. They don't even mind living on radioactive waste, so human skin poses no challenge whatsoever to their omnipresence. Skin is swarming with bacteria, and that's the way it's meant to be. There are on average one million bacteria on every square inch. Also present on our skin is sweat. Sweat contains a protein called cathelicidin, a natural antibiotic. It has potent anti-microbial activity and provides a barrier for protection against infection from pathogenic bacteria.[43] This has been described by researchers as an 'ancient and efficient innate defence mechanism',[44] which explains why skin infections are relatively rare considering our constant exposure to external pathogens.[45] Those of us who see no need for antibacterial hand washes, sprays and so on are not dying in droves.

We've got ourselves stuck in a loop and it's hard to see a way out. An exit strategy does exist, however, even though it is yet to form part of any public health pronouncement: accept that bacteria control us, despite our efforts to control them, and build up your immunity by looking after your invisible friends. Learn to love the life within.

Case History

Maggie was 33 years old, with a stressful job in publishing, coping with constipation, digestive discomfort (she could only manage very small meals), very low energy all the time, headaches, mild depression and recurrent thrush. She had seen her doctor frequently and was apparently quite healthy. Her diet wasn't too bad at all: there was salad and other green vegetables, but Maggie had a sweet tooth and was fond of sweetened yoghurts and refined carbohydrates such as pasta and pizza. She also rather liked white wine and drank regularly. Most worrying, though, was her antibiotic history: like so many people I see, she had a history of regular antibiotic intake, in her case because of recurrent cystitis. For over ten years she had taken around three courses a year (which is nothing, compared to some people I've seen).

I suggested a comprehensive parasitology test, but somehow we never got round to doing one. It wasn't really necessary, as it turned out. I was quite confident that underlying all her problems was a state of gut dysbiosis, quite probably with a yeast overgrowth.

I recommended cutting all sweet foods and most carbohydrates from her diet, other than porridge and, of course, fruit and vegetables. I developed a plan which was packed with plant foods high in fibre, including beans and lentils. Out went the alcohol as well.

I recommended a good basic multivitamin and -mineral and extra vitamin C to help strengthen Maggie's immune system. I also recommended a hefty dose of probiotics (combining both lactic acid bacteria, Bifidobacteria and fructo-oligosaccharides).

I saw Maggie three weeks later. She had stuck to the diet regime and was eating lots of live yoghurt with fresh fruit, lentils, chickpeas and other beans, green salads and other vegetables, nuts and oily fish. Her constipation and digestive discomfort (mainly flatulence and bloating) had completely gone, as had her regular headaches. Her energy levels had improved but were still not ideal, and she reported feeling 'stronger' and her depression had improved, although not vanished.

I decided that Maggie's dysbiosis was probably quite severe and that extra help was needed, so this time kept her diet the same but added in a few extra anti-fungal supplements – oregano oil and caprylic acid. She was to stay on the probiotics.

The third and final time I saw Maggie was four weeks later. With regard to her digestion, she said the changes were 'phenomenal'. In addition, her energy was now really good and her mild depression had lifted. In my notes I recorded that Maggie had commented that she 'felt like a normal human being'. Naturally I was as delighted as she was. I advised that she stay on her new dietary regime as much as possible but not to worry about the occasional blip, as I felt her immune system would now be able to cope. I also felt that occasional social drinking would do no harm, and suggested she stick with red wine. I'm glad to say, in the nicest possible way, that I never saw Maggie again.

FURTHER INVESTIGATIONS

If this chapter resonates with you, I strongly advise you to read the Solution 8 chapter straight away. Dysbiosis and leaky gut frequently (though not always) go hand in hand, and in order to have a healthy gut you may need to deal with both issues.

Solution 8
Healing a Leaky Gut

To many people the term 'leaky gut' suggests some implausible, alternative-leaning pseudo-science. Be that as it may, it is the name frequently used in place of the more technical nomenclature, 'intestinal permeability'. 'Intestinal permeability' may have more scientific gravitas than the slapstick 'leaky gut', but the latter is more visual, and the image of a colander-like gut that this term brings to mind is not entirely off the mark.

Leaky gut/intestinal permeability is a common – yet, in some rare cases, deadly – condition. Your intestines are lined with a single layer of cells whose job it is to create a barrier between the outside world and your insides. If this lining of cells becomes porous through damage, the barrier is compromised and mayhem ensues. I often liken having a leaky gut to having broken doors on the house, leaving you vulnerable to dangerous intruders.

Whenever I mention intestinal permeability to clients, friends or passers-by, virtually none of them has heard of it. The subject appears seldom to arise in the GP's surgery. Yet the scientific literature on leaky gut/intestinal permeability is vast, and the condition is well documented as a major cause of not only gut but whole-body symptoms.

ABOUT THE GUT LINING

As we saw in Solution 7, the gut has a dual role. First it must digest food and allow the passage of nutrients extracted from this digested matter into the blood. Secondly, the gut must act as a selective barrier, sifting out the undesirable contents of the gut and preventing them from spilling into the bloodstream. It is this second role which concerns us here.

The lining of the gut goes by a variety of names, including: intestinal mucosa, the mucous membrane and the mucosal barrier. Sometimes it is referred to as the *epithelium*, as it consists, extraordinarily, of just a single layer of cells. The sheet of cells which make up the epithelium are held together by what are termed 'tight junctions'. These tight junctions, which are made of proteins, work like intestinal 'bouncers', allowing in nutrients but barring harmful toxins, microorganisms, undigested food molecules and any foreign matter that has found its way into our food and drink.

WHAT IS LEAKY GUT SYNDROME?

The thin layer separating your internal body from the external world can, with alarming ease, become damaged and porous. Damage leads to irritation and inflammation, and as a result the tight junctions loosen up and microscopic holes arise, allowing larger molecules to pass through which ordinarily wouldn't make it. Pathogenic bacteria, toxic molecules and undigested food can all pass unchallenged into the bloodstream. When you consider some of the rubbish you may have eaten, or stuff you may even have swallowed by mistake, a leaky gut is an unnerving thought.

Symptoms of Leaky Gut

Almost everything circulating in the blood has access to the whole body. Consequently, symptoms of leaky gut may manifest anywhere, starting in the digestive system and ending anywhere you care to mention – the brain, the joints, the skin ... Typical symptoms of a leaky gut are, therefore, manifold and affect every bodily system. They include:

- bloating

- abdominal pain

- excessive abdominal gas

- constipation

- diarrhoea

- chronic joint pain

- poor immunity

- skin problems – acne, eczema, psoriasis, rashes

- fatigue

- fuzzy thinking

- poor memory and concentration

- mood swings

- anxiety

- depression

- recurrent thrush
- recurrent bladder infections.

WHAT HAPPENS WHEN YOU HAVE A LEAKY GUT

The above symptoms are the fall-out of intestinal damage. Intestinal damage arising from leaky gut has four main consequences: translocation of bacteria, inflammation, immune/allergic response and liver toxicity.

Translocation of Bacteria

This means that undesirable bacteria, which should ideally stay put in the gut, are able to move through the gut lining and into the bloodstream. With these bacteria comes endotoxin, which is the toxic substance released by the cell walls of pathogenic bacteria when they are destroyed. When endotoxin travels from the intestine to the circulation, it can initiate injury to the liver and other organs.[1]

Inflammation

One of the major characteristics of leaky gut syndrome is inflammation. Endotoxin from pathogenic bacteria and other substances can stimulate the inflammatory response. The role of inflammation is to clear up infection, but it can also give rise to pain and fatigue.

Immune and Allergic Response

The arrival of large molecules, endotoxin and infection caused by bacteria, parasites and fungi, via the gut lining, provokes the immune system into producing antibodies to fight off these foreign invaders (known as *antigens*). Partially digested food molecules are also perceived as alien, and their absorption through the gut lining can result in multiple food sensitivities – see Solution 1 chapter. Also produced by the immune system are proteins called *cytokines*, secreted in response to trauma or infection and which also fight antigens. Unfortunately, these cytokines can also cause the gut lining to become leaky.[2] Some cytokines are pro-inflammatory as part of an aggressive response to an antigen. Cytokines also alert white blood cells called lymphocytes to join in the fight.

People who have a genetic tendency to develop the classic allergic diseases – dermatitis (a form of eczema), asthma and hay fever – are known as *atopic*. In one study of this subject it was found that atopic people who also had irritable bowel syndrome were more likely to have increased intestinal permeability than IBS patients without atopic symptoms.[3] There is certainly plenty of literature which supports the finding that leaky gut appears to be the norm in atopic individuals. Interestingly, another study also found that not only is intestinal permeability present in all people who have adverse food reactions, there is also a statistically significant association between the severity of the symptoms of food sensitivity and the severity of the intestinal permeability.[4]

Inflammation is a common denominator in the many conditions caused or aggravated by leaky gut. Asthma is one such inflammatory condition. Leaky gut has already been linked to asthma in adults, and in one study of 32 asthmatic children, intestinal permeability was found to be significantly increased, compared with 32 non-asthmatic children.[5]

Liver Toxicity

The liver is normally a fine, efficient organ of detoxification, capable of filtering out the usual everyday detritus. However, the stuff that arrives in the blood from a leaky gut can be a challenge too far, and this extra burden means the liver has to process a great deal more than it would under healthy circumstances. Prolonged antibody response can also overwhelm the overworked liver. So what it can't cope with is sent back into circulation, where it ends up in connective tissue, joints, muscles and skin. The liver will also pass toxins to fat cells for storage (as described in Solution 5).

CONDITIONS ASSOCIATED WITH LEAKY GUT

Irritable Bowel Syndrome (IBS)

There is growing evidence that people with IBS also have increased intestinal permeability, and this intestinal permeability is thought to be a possible cause of IBS-associated inflammation.[6] The discovery that increased gut permeability and inflammation are found in people with IBS is a recent one.[7]

Coeliac Disease

Coeliac disease is a severe reaction to an allergen, namely the gluten component of certain grains. The absorption sites along the intestines – hair-like protrusions called villi and microvilli – are worn smooth, so food is not properly assimilated. Symptoms of coeliac disease include pain, diarrhoea and weight loss. Avoidance of gluten, found in wheat, rye, oats and barley, results in complete remission.

Intestinal permeability is a feature of coeliac disease, and avoidance of gluten allows the permeability of the gut to return to almost normal in the majority of coeliacs.[8] Although people with coeliac disease clearly have leaky gut, it is not known if leaky gut is a causal factor, a contributor to the disease, or the result of the disease.[9]

Inflammatory Bowel Disorder

People with IBD are known to have impaired gut barrier function[10] (for details of IBD, see page 146). Levels of inflammatory markers, cytokines, are raised in IBD, and these cytokines are known to cause the intestinal barrier to become leaky.[11] Crohn's disease is one of the main types of IBD. Although the cause of Crohn's disease remains unknown, what is known (at least as found in animal subjects), is that abnormal permeability is present *before* the disease occurs. In humans, increased gut permeability is commonly observed in people considered to be at high risk of developing Crohn's. Indeed, there is considerable data which support the hypothesis that there is a gut permeability abnormality in Crohn's disease, and that this abnormality plays a role in the initiation of the condition,[12] although which comes first – intestinal permeability or Crohn's disease – is still not fully established.[13]

Alcoholic Liver Disease

Alcohol can seriously damage the gut lining, and both alcoholic liver disease and fatty liver disease are associated with intestinal permeability. Having said that, only 30 per cent of alcoholics go on to develop chronic liver disease.[14] Increased intestinal permeability has been found in alcoholics with liver disease, but not in alcoholics without liver disease.[15] There has to be a reason for this, and experimental studies 'strongly suggest' that endotoxin – the toxin released from bacteria which translocate from the gut to the blood – is essential to the development of alcohol-related liver injury.[16] Endotoxin is also found in the blood of patients with alcoholic cirrhosis.[17] What this also means is that the key to whether or not an alcoholic develops liver disease may lie in whether or not he or she has a leaky gut, which is a sobering thought.

Depression

Depression is a highly complex condition and its causes are known to be multifactorial, but one potential cause is inflammation in the gut. Depression has been linked to altered levels of inflammatory cytokines, those chemicals released by the immune system in response to infection. This fascinating association has been investigated and it has been found that the toxic by-products produced by bad bacteria in the gut – endotoxin – play a role in the development of depression where there are increased levels of inflammatory cytokines.[18]

Chronic Fatigue Syndrome

People with chronic fatigue syndrome are known to have both intestinal permeability and dysbiosis (the overgrowth of unfriendly bacteria in the small intestine – see the Solution 7 chapter). They have also been shown to have increased levels of endotoxin.[19] Treating both dysbiosis and intestinal permeability has been shown to improve symptoms in people with both chronic fatigue and depression.[20]

Diabetes

There has long been a suspected link between the gut and development of type 1 diabetes, and increased gut permeability in patients with diabetes was first reported 20 years ago. More recent studies have confirmed that leaky gut occurs frequently in type 1 diabetes patients, whereas type 2 diabetes sufferers are more likely to have normal intestinal permeability.[21]

One particular, recent study set out to determine whether intestinal permeability actually helped cause type 1 diabetes or was secondary to the condition. Eighty-one people with either pre-clinical diabetes, new-onset diabetes or established type 1 diabetes were tested, and each one of them was found to have a leaky gut, a finding which led the researchers to conclude that leaky gut is already detectable before clinical onset of diabetes, and the gut is in some way involved in the development of the disease.[22]

Skin Disorders

The skin is a major organ of detoxification and a convenient dumping site for the overburdened liver dealing with the fall-out of a leaky gut. So it is hardly surprising that various skin conditions, especially those which involve inflammation, are associated with gut permeability. In a study of 18 people with dermatitis herpetiformis (a blistering skin disease associated with coeliac disease), all participants were found to have increased intestinal permeability. It is also thought that damage to the gut lining is involved in the development of atopic dermatitis, a form of eczema.[23]

Arthritic Conditions

Arthritis has long been associated with abnormalities of the gut and is in fact a painful manifestation of a number of digestive disorders, including inflammatory bowel disorder (arthritis occurs in up to half of patients with IBD), coeliac disease and parasitic infestation.[24] Because arthritic symptoms tend to improve when the digestive disorder is treated, it is thought that these two clinical entities are related even though the mechanism of the relationship is not fully understood.

Three types of arthritis – ankylosing spondylitis, reactive arthritis and psoriatic arthritis – belong to a group of arthritic conditions called the spondyloarthropathy group. Up to two-thirds of patients with spondyloarthropathies have been found to have sub-clinical gut inflammation.

Ankylosing spondylitis is a chronic inflammatory disease characterized by back pain and spine rigidity. Leaky gut has been associated with ankylosing spondylitis for decades, though it has in the past been unclear if the leaky gut was due to the condition itself or its treatment. Recently, however, it has been found that patients with ankylosing spondylitis have a primary defect in intestinal permeability.[25]

Reactive arthritis may occur after contracting some kind of parasitic infection, especially salmonella, shigella, yersinia, campylobacter and *Endolimax nana*. Joint symptoms – the knee, ankle, wrist and sacroiliac joints – arise within two to three weeks of developing diarrhoea.[26]

Sepsis Syndrome

Sepsis is an infection which has spread throughout the body, in the blood, and is often referred to as either blood poisoning or septicaemia. There are around 31,000 cases of severe sepsis a year in England and Wales, and approximately 30–50 per cent of those affected will die because of the infection. There is, according to research, 'ample evidence' linking gut barrier dysfunction to multi-organ system failure in sepsis.[27] Indeed, the scientific literature on the subject is awash with evidence pointing to a significant association between sepsis and leaky gut. It is easy to imagine how this occurs: dangerous toxins enter the blood via a porous gut, and once there are free to circulate around the body, stopping off anywhere en route.

Pancreatitis

People with acute pancreatitis (inflammation of the pancreas which can cause severe abdominal pain) have been found to have significantly high levels of endotoxin, the toxin secreted by pathogenic bacteria. They have also been found to have significantly higher levels of inflammatory cytokines and increased intestinal permeability, compared to people without the condition.[28]

WHAT CAUSES LEAKY GUT?

Like most of the subjects covered in this book, the cause of leaky gut is not a conveniently simple, readily identifiable one. Leaky gut is a complex condition with myriad possible causes. Any irritation to the gut lining can make permeability worse, and irritation arises from a number of sources, the main ones being: dysbiosis, allergens, certain medications, alcohol and free radicals.

Dysbiosis/Parasitic Infection

Microscopic bugs are known to damage the gut lining and produce toxins that exacerbate irritation and increase gut permeability.[29] Yeasts such as candida are able to burrow their way into the intestinal lining. Other parasites also cause irritation to the gut lining, making it more permeable: *Blastocystis hominis*, giardia, *Helicobacter pylori*, salmonella and shigella are all known intestinal offenders. However, one of the most significant offenders is thought to be campylobacter. Irritable bowel syndrome develops in up to 25 per cent of patients following infection with campylobacter. In a study of one such group of patients it was found that gut permeability was also significantly elevated.[30]

If you have read Solution 7 on dysbiosis you may have noticed by now that a link between parasitic infection, irritable bowel syndrome (IBS) and leaky gut is clearly emerging. Between 6 and 17 per cent of IBS patients claim that their symptoms began with a gut infection. This claim is supported by clinical tests which have shown that between 4 and 31 per cent of people develop IBS following bacterial gastroenteritis. IBS has been found to develop following infection with campylobacter, salmonella and shigella. This is not a new, startling revelation: the development of IBS after contracting a parasite infection is a phenomenon that was first described as long ago as 1962.[31]

Medications

A number of drugs are known to disrupt the gut significantly. These include chemotherapy drugs, but none more notoriously so than non-steroidal anti-inflammatory drugs (NSAIDs) which are known to increase gut permeability within 24 hours of taking them. The best-known NSAIDs are probably aspirin and ibuprofen. In tests, around two-thirds of NSAID users have been shown to have intestinal inflammation and increased gut permeability.[32]

Chronic Stress

The brain–gut interaction is both fascinating and poorly understood. There is, however, growing scientific interest in the effects of psychological stress on the intestinal barrier. The data emerging from studies suggests that there are signalling pathways linking the central nervous system and cells of the intestinal barrier. It is difficult to monitor the effects of stress on the human gut lining, but animal studies have found that stress increases the passage through the intestinal barrier of small molecules produced by bacteria, as well as large molecules in the form of undigested proteins.[33]

Alcohol

In addition to its better known misdemeanours, alcohol can also promote the growth of pathogenic bacteria, and the result of this is endotoxin, the toxic substance created from the cell walls of bacteria that travels to the liver and elsewhere. Furthermore, when bacteria metabolize alcohol, the result is an accumulation of the chemical acetaldehyde (popularly believed to be the cause of hangovers) which increases intestinal permeability.

Free Radicals

The oxygen used by the body to produce energy results in the production of highly reactive chemicals called free radicals. This process is called oxidative stress. Free radicals are also created by smoking, pollution and certain cooking methods such as barbecuing. These free radicals can be very damaging to body cells, and unhindered free radicals are implicated in many diseases, including cancer and heart disease. Oxidative stress is a well-known cause of intestinal permeability, disrupting the tight junctions between cells and compromising the gut barrier.[34]

HAVE YOU GOT A LEAKY GUT?

Quite simply, without testing it is impossible to know the answer to this question for sure, although it is possible to build a strong case based on symptoms and history alone. A leaky gut test will not only tell you if you have it, but, if so, how badly. And if you know that much, you have an indication of just how long it will take to heal.

Before you make any decisions, ask yourself the following questions:

• Do you have dysbiosis, or suspect that you may have?

• Have you had a parasitic infection?

- Do you smoke? Smoking is free-radical hell.

- Do you drink alcohol regularly?

- Do you have a history of stress?

- Have you taken NSAIDs, such as aspirin, regularly?

- Do you eat a low-fibre, low-antioxidant diet? See page 191 for details of antioxidant foods.

Answering 'yes' to any of the above means that it is possible that you may have a leaky gut, and answering 'yes' to more than one increases that likelihood, especially if you have one or more symptoms of gut permeability.

WHAT TO DO NOW

- First, read Solution 7 on dysbiosis. If you have overgrowth of pathogenic bacteria, or a yeast or parasitic infection, you have to deal with this first, as these are a major cause of leaky gut.

- Next, visit your GP to ensure that you do not have an underlying intestinal disorder such as coeliac disease, ulcerative colitis and so on.

- Thirdly, decide whether or not to test for leaky gut. I advise that if you feel you would like to do this you do so with the guidance of a nutritional therapist who will be able to interpret the results and devise a healing programme to suit you.

Testing for Leaky Gut

There is a very simple urine test used in medical laboratories which indicates whether or not your intestinal wall is leaky. It is sometimes known as the lactulose/mannitol test. To do the test, you drink a solution containing lactulose and mannitol. These are harmless water-soluble sugar molecules which the body does not metabolize so they pass easily through the body. Mannitol is a small molecule, readily absorbed by the healthy digestion system, so serves as a good indicator of healthy absorption. Lactulose, however, is a larger molecule, and because less than 1 per cent of the dose taken should pass through the gut lining, it serves as a good marker of permeability.

After drinking the solution you collect your urine over a period of 6 hours, and draw off a sample. Low levels of mannitol indicate malabsorption. Elevated levels of both lactulose and mannitol are indicative of increased permeability, or leaky gut. The ratio between the two sugars is also significant. A normal lactulose/ mannitol ratio in urine should be less than 0.03. Anything higher than this suggests excessive permeability.

HEALING THE LEAKY GUT

How long it takes to heal a leaky gut depends on the severity of the damage. From experience I would say that the process takes at least 2 months and may take up to a year. There are various approaches, which are all helpful and which I have outlined below. There are no pharmaceutical medicines available to heal intestinal permeability, which may explain why GPs do not as a rule treat this condition.

Probiotics

The friendly bacteria in your gut, with which you are now familiar, are key not just to healthy intestines but also to a healthy gut lining. Probiotics, when used therapeutically, appear to work in several ways. They compete with pathogens for adhesion to the intestinal lining and at the same time stimulate the gut's immune system to produce anti-inflammatory substances.[35] Lactic acid bacteria have been shown to prevent free-radical disruption of tight junctions and to preserve barrier function.[36] In children with atopic dermatitis, lactic acid bacteria have been found to significantly decrease the frequency of gastrointestinal symptoms. The children who were studied were also shown, through lactulose/mannitol testing, to have improved intestinal permeability after taking probiotics. Skin symptoms also improved from taking lactic acid bacteria, leading the researchers to conclude that impairment of the intestinal barrier may in some way be involved in the development of atopic dermatitis.[37]

It is important to establish a healthy gut lining as early as possible. Children are much more prone to allergies, possibly because their guts have not fully matured. Children with cow's milk allergy have been found to have increased permeability.[38] Breastfeeding is important in establishing a healthy gut lining, as it increases levels of infection-fighting antibodies and levels of beneficial flora.

Adults, on the other hand, are more prone to the various forms of inflammatory bowel disorder. In a study of 34 patients with Crohn's disease who were give either probiotics (*Saccharomyces boulardii*) or placebo, intestinal permeability was measured before, during and at the end of 3 months of treatment. At the end of the study, the Crohn's patients taking a placebo were found to have increased gut permeability, whereas those taking the probiotics showed the opposite – that is, an improvement in gut integrity.[39] Gut integrity was not fully restored, however, suggesting that in cases of Crohn's, at least, the healing process may take longer than 3 months.

Glutamine

Glutamine is a non-essential amino acid, meaning that the body is able to make it. It is in fact the most abundant amino acid in the body. It is mainly obtained from the diet, meat being one of the best sources. It provides energy to muscle and helps build tissue. In large doses it has been shown to have remarkable therapeutic properties. Glutamine is the primary fuel used by the cells of the intestine to repair itself. Along with probiotics, it is the most effective product available for mending a leaky gut. Its therapeutic benefits have been well documented and it has been shown to improve and protect intestinal barrier function.[40] In practice, many of my clients have commented on how much better they feel soon after starting to take glutamine.

Many studies have been carried out on the therapeutic use of glutamine in people who have developed intestinal permeability due to different causes. Glutamine is effective in people whose gut permeability has been induced by taking NSAIDs.[41] It is also useful in the treatment of people with infections in parts of the body other than the digestive system, as it is thought that it may help prevent pathogenic bacteria and their toxic by-products from moving from the gut to the blood.[42] Patients who are critically ill with an infection often have increased intestinal permeability, and glutamine has been shown to improve gut integrity in those patients.[43]

Aloe Vera Juice

Probiotics and glutamine appear to actively heal the gut. Other substances work by reducing inflammation. One such substance is aloe vera juice. Aloe is both an antioxidant and anti-inflammatory agent, and for this reason is thought to be therapeutic in the treatment of inflammatory bowel disorder.[44] It has also been found to improve the symptoms of ulcerative colitis significantly, compared to placebo.[45]

Zinc

Zinc is a trace element widely found in meat, fish and seafood and also in wholegrains, nuts and seeds. It plays many roles in the body and is involved in all protein structures. It is crucial for wound-healing, so it is not surprising that it is important in maintaining and healing the intestinal lining. In animal studies, zinc has been shown to enhance the function of tight junctions, and in humans, zinc supplementation has been shown to preserve intestinal permeability in patients with Crohn's disease.[46]

What to Eat

- First, consider *how* you eat. One unfortunate consequence of leaky gut is the passage of undigested food through the gut barrier. Therefore, the more you chew your food before swallowing, the better digested it will be by the time it reaches your small intestine, and the less likely therefore to cause a reaction.

- Avoid foods to which you have a sensitivity. If you suspect that something you are eating is causing a reaction, but have not yet identified the offender(s), read the Solution 1 chapter, which discusses food intolerances.

- Follow a diet which favours the friendly bacteria in your gut and therefore reduces your risk of developing intestinal permeability – see page 166, Solution 7 for details of this diet.

- In addition to foods which feed friendly bacteria, you need to incorporate foods high in antioxidants and phytonutrients and low in free radicals. Antioxidants are natural plant chemicals which disarm those dangerous free radicals, which, as previously mentioned, are one of the main causes of intestinal permeability.

Antioxidants and Phytonutrients

Oxygen is a highly reactive chemical in the body, and free oxidizing radicals attack the DNA of the cells, causing damage and affecting cell replication. To the rescue come antioxidants, the best known of which are perhaps the vitamins C and E, the mineral selenium, and the vitamin A precursor, beta carotene. However there are hundreds if not thousands of antioxidant chemicals in foods, and these are also known as phytochemicals.

The best sources of antioxidant nutrients and phytochemicals are plant foods, namely fruits, vegetables, legumes, nuts, seeds and wholegrains. The best sources of vitamin C are the berry fruits (blueberries, strawberries, and other berries), kiwi fruit, citrus fruits and potatoes. Vitamin E is often found together with selenium in nuts and seeds, especially pumpkin seeds, cashew nuts, walnuts and Brazil nuts. Nuts are also an especially good source of the antioxidant enzyme glutathione.

Phytochemicals are broadly categorized into two groups: carotenoids and polyphenols. The best-known carotenoid is beta carotene, as found in carrots. Other excellent sources of carotenoids include sweet potato, pumpkin, squash, yellow peppers and other orange or red plant foods, such as tomatoes. Dark leafy greens such as spinach and kale are rich sources of carotenoids, too, as are the famous cruciferous vegetables (which I can barely stop myself from evangelizing about at every opportunity): cabbage, cauliflower, broccoli, Brussels sprouts, curly kale, spinach.

The best-known polyphenols are the flavonoids, powerful antioxidants which are also potent anti-inflammatory agents. They are found in a wide variety of plant foods, and some are easily identifiable by their colour – deep reds, purples and blues are the mark of a flavonoid. These include those vitamin C-rich berries (especially blueberries and blackberries), plums, grapes and red onion. Other flavonoids are found in soya beans, soya products and citrus fruits, pulses and cocoa. Other polyphenol-rich sources worthy of mention are green tea, certain herbs (especially rosemary and thyme), turmeric and mushrooms – in particular shiitake, maitake and reishi.

Essential Fats

Include plenty of essential fats in your diet. Essential fats are powerfully anti-inflammatory and are required to help repair damage to the gut lining – see page 74 for good sources of these fats.

Anti-inflammatory Foods

Consume plenty of foods that are known to have anti-inflammatory properties, including oily fish (those good fats again), ginger, fennel seeds, garlic, slippery elm tea, oregano, oats. Although these foods are known for their anti-inflammatory properties, the only one which has been shown to affect intestinal permeability directly is, to my knowledge, oats – giving oats to rats has been shown to reverse induced gut leakiness, thought it is not known how.[47]

Proteins

Ensure adequate protein, especially zinc-rich foods. Oily fish is ideal because it contains zinc, protein *and* anti-inflammatory fatty acids.

Case History

For my final case I thought I'd describe my own health issues, which I eventually came to clear up through nutritional therapy after a history of totally ineffectual medical treatments.

Throughout my teens and twenties I was plagued with digestive symptoms – at times quite severe irritable bowel accompanied by some extraordinary bloating. The internal chaos I endured was reflected in my skin – itchy rashes and spots were the bane of my life. Of course at that stage I was a nutritional philistine and had no idea that there was an association between my bowel disorder and my skin problems. What shocks me now is that neither did any of the doctors or specialists I consulted for both conditions. I took lots of medications for IBS, which had no effect at all. I saw a skin specialist in Harley Street who gave me antibiotics for my acne, which were also ineffective. I also visited a Chinese herbalist, on whose advice I brewed up various foul-tasting concoctions, which had a sum effect of zero.

To cut a long story short, once I started studying nutrition it became clear to me that diet was almost certainly key to restoring my overall health. I arranged for a laboratory to carry out a comprehensive parasitology test, and sure enough this revealed I had dysbiosis and the parasite *B. hominis* (as described in the Solution 7 chapter). I followed the appropriate diet and took probiotics and herbal medicine. My symptoms improved enormously – but not completely, so I knew I had to go a step further and do the intestinal permeability test. The results were as I'd suspected. Lactulose levels were virtually off the page, mannitol was only just within the normal range, and the lactulose/mannitol ratio was also in the red. I had a very leaky gut.

One thing I have always observed with my clients who choose to undergo tests is that, no matter how bad the results, they are always relieved finally to know what it is that is causing their symptoms. That is exactly how I felt. All those years of pain, embarrassment and elasticated waistbands were coming to an end. I followed the appropriate dietary steps to heal a leaky gut and took a level teaspoon of glutamine powder, twice a day. The glutamine was effective from the start – I felt as if a wild beast within had been tamed. My skin cleared up. I concentrated on anti-inflammatory foods, took aloe vera, made lemon and ginger teas every day and avoided alcohol most of the time. Nearly 20 years later I still feel utterly relieved that I no longer endure the daily torment of IBS.

FURTHER INVESTIGATIONS

As already discussed in this chapter, you should also read the Solution 1 (food sensitivities) and Solution 7 (dysbiosis) chapters if you have, or suspect you have, a leaky gut. If stress is a real issue in your life, or has been for prolonged periods, you may also benefit from reading the Solution 3 (adrenal fatigue) chapter. As we've seen, chronic stress can be a causative factor in the development of leaky gut.

Meal Ideas

By now you hopefully have a fairly clear idea of what you need to do to get rid of all those tedious yet tenacious symptoms. But what do you eat? In each chapter I've told you what individual foods to eat, but the question now is how to transform those individual food items into a meal.

I have always given my clients meal ideas rather than recipes because I want them to understand not just what to eat but *how* to eat for their health requirements. This is intended to be a practical book, and on a practical level you are unlikely to follow recipes three times a day. Many of the components of these meal ideas are interchangeable and can be adapted to suit your needs and tastes. What's more, many meals can also be easily assembled either at home or in the workplace, with little or minimal cooking.

Please note that Solution 1 is not included in the tables below – obviously this is because suitability depends on what you are sensitive to, or which foods you are testing. You can adapt most of these ideas to suit your food sensitivities.

POINTS TO REMEMBER

Choose organic wherever possible, especially when it comes to fatty foods. In Solution 5 you read about how fatty foods tend to be high in toxins. Organic, free-range eggs are superior to eggs from non-organic, indoor-reared birds because they are richer in essential fatty acids.

Nut butters, other than peanut butter, are usually available from health food stores. Tinned foods are quick, easy and convenient but aim to avoid those with a plastic lining, as this may contain xenoestrogens (see Solution 5). Tinned tuna is a good source of protein but not fatty acids as these are destroyed during the canning process.

The meal ideas below are divided into different sections for breakfast, lunch and dinner. Each meal option has either one, two or three stars indicating how suitable it is for the problem addressed in each Solution chapter.

BREAKFAST IDEAS

Plain bio (live) yoghurt with any or all of the following: chopped or puréed fruit, prunes, a sprinkling of chopped nuts and seeds, flaked almonds, desiccated coconut

Suitable for Solution	2	3	4	5	6	7	8
	***	***	**	***	**	***	***

Live natural soya yoghurt with any of the above additions

Suitable for Solution	2	3	4	5	6	7	8
	***	***	**	***	**	***	***

Stewed apples with prunes and prune juice with natural live yoghurt

Suitable for Solution	2	3	4	5	6	7	8
	**	**	*	**	*	***	***

Sugar-free, wholegrain muesli (high nut/seed content) with milk

Suitable for Solution	2	3	4	5	6	7	8
	**	**	**	**	**	**	**

Oatcakes with cashew or hazelnut butter

Suitable for Solution	2	3	4	5	6	7	8
	***	***	**	**	**	***	***

Oatcakes dipped in live natural yoghurt

Suitable for Solution	2	3	4	5	6	7	8
	***	***	*	**	**	***	***

Porridge with milk and fresh fruit/prunes/nuts and seeds

Suitable for Solution	2	3	4	5	6	7	8
	***	***	**	**	**	***	***

Fruit salad or puréed mixed fruits with nuts and seeds (pumpkin, linseed, sunflower, sesame)

Suitable for Solution	2	3	4	5	6	7	8
	**	**	**	***	*	***	***

Poached/scrambled eggs, grilled tomatoes, mushrooms, sugar-free baked beans

Suitable for Solution	2	3	4	5	6	7	8
	***	***	**	**	**	**	**

Boiled/poached/scrambled egg on wholemeal rye toast

Suitable for Solution	2	3	4	5	6	7	8
	***	***	**	*	*	*	*

Kippers with tomatoes and mushrooms

Suitable for Solution	2	3	4	5	6	7	8
	***	***	***	**	**	**	**

Kedgeree – wholegrain rice with boiled egg and fish (undyed smoked haddock) and peas

Suitable for Solution	2	3	4	5	6	7	8
	**	**	*	**	**	**	**

Scrambled eggs with smoked wild salmon on wholemeal toast with grilled tomatoes

Suitable for Solution	2	3	4	5	6	7	8
	***	***	***	**	**	**	**

Turkish-style breakfast – boiled egg, sheep's cheese, tomatoes, olives, wholemeal bread

Suitable for Solution	2	3	4	5	6	7	8
	***	***	**	*	**	**	**

Boiled egg and wholemeal toast

Suitable for Solution	2	3	4	5	6	7	8
	**	**	**	*	**	**	**

Half a grapefruit; wholemeal toast with cashew/hazelnut nut butter

Suitable for Solution	2	3	4	5	6	7	8
	**	**	**	**	*	**	**

LUNCH AND DINNER IDEAS

Wholemeal sandwiches with a protein filling – meat, tuna, egg or cheese – but in addition stuffed with green leafy salad leaves such as rocket or watercress. Alternatively, or in addition, slice up half an avocado and add that.

Suitable for Solution	2	3	4	5	6	7	8
	**	**	*	**	*	**	**

Mixed bean salad (you can buy tins of mixed beans) with sliced tomato, red onion, marinated tofu and sweetcorn with a virgin olive oil dressing

Suitable for Solution	2	3	4	5	6	7	8
	***	***	*	***	**	***	***

Greek salad – olives, feta cheese, sliced red onion, tomatoes, red pepper, salad leaves

Suitable for Solution	2	3	4	5	6	7	8
	***	***	*	***	**	***	***

Egg and potato salad (new pots; keep skin on) with cucumber and spring onion, mayo

Suitable for Solution	2	3	4	5	6	7	8
	**	**	**	**	**	**	**

Bulgur wheat/barley salad with mixed vegetables and nuts, e.g. cashews and Brazils

Suitable for Solution	2	3	4	5	6	7	8
	**	**	**	***	**	***	***

Vegetable and bean soup with grated cheddar on top and wholegrain bread roll

Suitable for Solution	2	3	4	5	6	7	8
	***	***	*	***	**	***	***

Omelette with broccoli

Suitable for Solution	2	3	4	5	6	7	8
	***	***	**	***	**	***	***

Hummus with sticks of raw carrot, celery and green/red peppers

Suitable for Solution	2	3	4	5	6	7	8
	***	***	*	***	**	***	***

Avocado, tomato and mozzarella salad with fresh basil leaves and virgin olive oil

Suitable for Solution	2	3	4	5	6	7	8
	***	***	*	**	**	***	***

Prawns and avocado with vinaigrette dressing

Suitable for Solution	2	3	4	5	6	7	8
	***	***	*	**	***	**	**

Baked potato with cottage cheese, hummus, tuna/mayo/sweetcorn mix, sugar-free baked beans

Suitable for Solution	2	3	4	5	6	7	8
	*	*	*	**	*	**	**

Smoked mackerel fillet (peppered or plain) with green salad or spinach

Suitable for Solution	2	3	4	5	6	7	8
	***	***	***	***	***	***	***

Oily fish (baked or grilled) – mackerel, sardines, wild salmon/trout, herring or tuna with bean salad, mixed vegetables or green salad

Suitable for Solution	2	3	4	5	6	7	8
	***	***	***	***	***	***	***

Chicken leg/breast or other unprocessed meat with creamed sweet potato and carrot mix or dhal and broccoli/Brussels sprouts/ spinach

Suitable for Solution	2	3	4	5	6	7	8
	***	***	*	***	**	***	***

Stir-fry vegetables with tofu, seaweed, wholegrain rice

Suitable for Solution	2	3	4	5	6	7	8
	**	**	*	***	***	**	**

Prawn curry with lots of mixed vegetables and wholegrain basmati rice

Suitable for Solution	2	3	4	5	6	7	8
	**	**	*	**	***	**	**

Chili con carne served with leafy green salad/broccoli and/or dhal

Suitable for Solution	2	3	4	5	6	7	8
	***	***	*	***	**	***	***

Stir-fried bean sprouts and other vegetables (carrots, peppers, onions) with seafood cocktail

Suitable for Solution	2	3	4	5	6	7	8
	***	***	*	**	***	***	***

Home-made bean burger with salad

Suitable for Solution	2	3	4	5	6	7	8
	***	***	*	***	**	***	***

Roast joint of beef/lamb/pork with roasted potatoes/dhal, Brussels sprouts and carrots

Suitable for Solution	2	3	4	5	6	7	8
	**	**	*	***	**	**	**

Wholemeal quiche with salad

Suitable for Solution	2	3	4	5	6	7	8
	***	***	**	**	**	***	***

Bean casserole topped with grated cheddar

Suitable for Solution	2	3	4	5	6	7	8
	***	***	*	***	**	***	***

Ratatouille with chicken

Suitable for Solution	2	3	4	5	6	7	8
	***	***	*	**	**	***	***

Mixed grilled veg (aubergines, peppers, red onion) on grilled polenta topped with melted goat's cheese

Suitable for Solution	2	3	4	5	6	7	8
	**	**	*	**	**	**	**

Prawns and steamed white fish (cod, haddock), flaked with peas and wholegrain rice. served with salad

Suitable for Solution	2	3	4	5	6	7	8
	**	**	*	**	***	***	***

Resources

TESTS

Genova Diagnostics Europe
Tel: 020 8336 7750
www.gdx.uk.net
Adrenal stress profile
Comprehensive parasitology
IgG 88-food panel (food intolerances)
Intestinal permeability assessment
Total thyroid screen

YorkTest Laboratories
0800 4582052
www.yorktest.com
email: customercare@yorktest.com
Foodscreen 113 food intolerance test

The Doctors Laboratory
020 7307 7373
tdl@tdlpathology.com
Urinary iodine

THERAPIES

British Association for Applied Nutrition and Nutritional Therapy (BANT)
www.bant.org.uk
08706 061284
e-mail: theadministrator@bant.org.uk

Association of Reflexologists
www.aor.org.uk

The British Acupuncture Council
www.acupuncture.org.uk
020 8735 0400

The British Herbal Medicine Association
www.bhma.info
0845 680 1134
e-mail: secretary@bhma.info

References

SOLUTION 1

1.   Atkinson, W., Sheldon, T. A., Shaath, N. and Whorwell, P. J. (2004). 'Food elimination based on IgG antibodies in irritable bowel syndrome: a randomised controlled trial', *Gut* 53: 1459-64
2.   Shanahan, M. D. and Whorwell P. J. (2005). 'IgG mediated food intolerance in irritable bowel syndrome: A real phenomenon or an epiphenomenon? ', *The American Journal of Gastroenterology* 100(7): 1558-59
3.   Hardman, G. and Hart, G. (2007). 'Dietary advice based on food-specific IgG results', *Nutrition and Food Science* 37(1): 16-23
4.   Holford, P. and Braly, J. (2005). *Hidden Food Allergies*. London: Piatkus
5.   The British Nutrition Foundation. *Food allergy and intolerance*. www.nutrition.org.uk accessed 20 March 2008
6.   Weinsier, R. L. and Krumdieck, C. L. (2000). 'Dairy foods and bone health: examination of the evidence', *American Journal of Clinical Nutrition* 72(3): 681-89

SOLUTION 2

1.   Pinhas-Hamiel, O. and Zeitler, P. (2005). 'The global spread of type 2 diabetes mellitus in children and adolescents', *Journal of Pediatrics* 146(5): 693-700
2.   PatientPlus UK. Insulin Resistance – syndrome X. www.patient. co.uk accessed May 2008
3.   Black, P. H. (2003). 'The inflammatory response is an integral part

of the stress response: Implications for atherosclerosis, insulin resistance, type 2 diabetes and metabolic syndrome X', *Brain, Behaviour and Immunity* 17(5): 350-64

4.   Natali, A. and Ferrannini, E. (2004). 'Hypertension, insulin resistance and the metabolic syndrome', *Endocrinology and Metabolism Clinics* 33(2)

5.   Cubeddu, L. X. and Hoffmann, I. S. (2002). 'Insulin resistance and upper-normal glucose levels in hypertension: a review', *Journal of Human Hypertension* 16 (Supp 1) S52-S55

6.   Kernan W. N. *et al.* (2002). 'Insulin resistance and risk for stroke', *Neurology* 59: 809-15

7.   Dunaif, A. (1997). 'Insulin resistance and the polycystic ovary syndrome: Mechanism and implications for pathogenesis', *Endocrine Reviews* 18(6): 774-800

8.   Watson, G. S. and Craft, S. (2003). 'The role of insulin resistance in the pathogenesis of Alzheimer's disease: Implications for treatment. Review article', *CNS Drugs* 17(1): 27-45

9.   Giovannucci, E. (2003). 'Nutrition, insulin, insulin-like growth factors and cancer', *Hormonal Metabolism Research* 35 (11-12): 694-704

10.   Rizkalla, S. W., Bellisle, F. and Slama, G. (2002). 'Health benefits of low glycaemic index foods, such as pulses, in diabetic patients and healthy individuals', *British Journal of Nutrition* 88(Supp 3): S255-S262

11.   Henriksen, E. J. (2002). 'Exercise effects of muscle insulin. Invited review: Effects of acute exercise and exercise training on insulin resistance', *Journal of Applied Physiology* 93(2): 788-96

SOLUTION 3

1.   Health and Safety Executive (www.hse.gov.uk) accessed May 2008

2.   British Association for Counselling and Psychotherapy (2005). *Insomniac Britain: Does anybody sleep here any more?* www.bacp. co.uk

3. BBC (2003). *Road rage hits most drivers*. www.news.bbc.co.uk Wednesday, 13 August

4. Tsigos, C. and Chrousos, G. P. (2002). 'Hypothalamic-pituitary-adrenal axis, neuroendocrine factors and stress', *Journal of Psychosomatic Research* 53: 865-71

5. Holtorf, K. (2008). 'Diagnosis and treatment of hypothalamic-pituitary-adrenal (HPA) axis dysfunction in patients with chronic fatigue syndrome (CFS) and fibromyalgia (FM)', *Journal of Chronic Fatigue Syndrome* 14(3): 59-88(30)

6. Ibid.

7. Tsigos and Chrousos, op cit.

8. Heim, C., Ehlert, U. and Hellhammer, D. H. (2000). 'The potential role of hypocortisolism in the pathophysiology of stress-related bodily disorders', *Psychoneuroendocrinology* 25: 1-35

9. Nieminen, L. R. G., Makino, K. K., Mehta, N. *et al.* (2006). 'Relationship between omega-3 fatty acids and plasma neuroactive steroids in alcoholism, depression and controls', *Prostaglandins, Leukotrienes and Essential Fatty Acids* 75(4-5): 309-14

10. Delarue, J., Matzinger, O., Binnert, C. *et al.* (2003). 'Fish oil prevents the adrenal activation elicited by mental stress in healthy men', *Diabetes Metabolism* 29: 289-95

SOLUTION 4

1. Simopoulos, A. P. (2008). 'The importance of the omega-6/omega-3 fatty acid ratio in cardiovascular disease and other chronic diseases', *Experimental Biology and Medicine* 233: 674-88

2. Stender, S. and Dyerberg, J. (2004). 'Influence of trans-fatty acids on health', *Annals of Nutrition and Metabolism* 48: 61-66

3. Slattery, M.L., Benson, J. *et al.* (2004). 'Trans-fatty acids and colon cancer', *Nutrition and cancer* 39(2): 170-75

4. King, I. B., Kristal, A. R. *et al.* (2005). 'Serum trans-fatty acids are associated with risk of prostate cancer in β-carotene and retinol efficacy trial', *Cancer Epidemiology Biomarkers and Prevention* 14: 988-92

5. Ibid.
6. Simopoulos (2008) op cit.
7. Ibid.
8. Ibid.
9. Ibid.
10. Simopoulos, A. P. (2004). 'Omega-6/omega-3 essential fatty acid ratio and chronic diseases', *Food Reviews International* 20(1): 77-90
11. Simopoulos, A. P. (2002). 'The importance of the ratio of omega-6/ omega-3 essential fatty acids', *Biomedicine and Pharmacotherapy* 56(8): 365-79
12. Calder, P. C. and Zurier, R. B. (2001). 'Polyunsaturated fatty acids and rheumatoid arthritis', *Current Opinion in Clinical Nutrition and Metabolic Care* 4(2): 115-21
13. Simopoulos (2002) op cit.
14. Crawford, M. and Marsh, D. (1995). *Nutrition and Evolution.* Connecticut: Keats Publishing Inc.
15. Ibid.
16. Scientific Advisory Committee on Nutrition (2004). *Advice on fish consumption: benefits and risks.* London: TSO
17. Food Standards Agency (2002). *Survey of Dioxins and Dioxin-like PCBs in Fish Oil Supplements.* Food Survey Information Sheet (Number 26/02)
18. SACN (2004) op cit.
19. Oken, E. *et al.* (2005). 'Maternal Fish Consumption, Hair Mercury, and Infant Cognition in a U.S. Cohort', *Environmental Health Pespectives* 113(10): 1376-80
20. Richardson, A. J. and Montgomery, P. (2005). 'The Oxford-Durham study: A randomized, controlled trial of dietary supplementation with fatty acids in children with developmental coordination disorder', *Pediatrics* 115(5): 1360-66
21. Food Standards Agency (2002) op cit.
22. SACN (2004) op cit.
23. Ibid.
24. Craig, R. and Mindell, J. (eds), *Health Survey for England 2006.* 'Cardiovascular disease and risk factors. The Information Centre'

25. Morris, M. C. *et al.* (2005). 'Fish Consumption and Cognitive Decline with Age in a Large Community Study', *Archives of Neurology* 62: 1-5

26. Boelsma, E., Hendriks, H. F. J. and Roza, L. (2001). 'Nutritional skin care: health effects of micronutrients and fatty acids', *American Journal of Clinical Nutrition* 73: 853-64

27. Miljanović, B., Trivedi, K. A. *et al.* (2005). 'The relationship between dietary n-3 and n-6 fatty acids and clinically diagnosed dry eye syndrome', *American Journal of Clinical Nutrition* 82(4): 887-93

28. Ibid.

29. Zamaria, N. (2004). 'Alteration of polyunsaturated fatty acid status and metabolism in health and disease', *Reproduction Nutrition Development* 44: 273-82

30. Maes, M., Mihaylova, I. and Leunis, J. C. (2005). 'In chronic fatigue syndrome, the decreased levels of omega-3 polyunsaturated fatty acids are related to lowered serum zinc and defects in T cell activation', *Neuroendocrinology Letters* 26(6): 745-51

31. Freeman, M. P. (2000). 'Omega-3 fatty acids in psychiatry: A review', *Annals of Clinical Psychiatry* 12(3): 159-65

32. Mental Health Foundation (2006). *Feeding Minds. The Impact of Food on Mental Health.* London: The Mental Health Foundation

33. Ibid.

SOLUTION 5

1. Abraham, G. E. (1983). 'Nutritional factors in the etiology of the premenstrual tension syndromes', *Journal of Reproductive Medicine* 28(7): 446-64

2. Lee, J. R. (1996). *What Your Doctor May Not Tell You About Menopause.* New York. Warner.

3. Cancer Research UK www.cancerresearch.org accessed September 2009.

4. Ibid.

5. Ibid.

6. Ibid.

7.   Ibid.
8.   Ibid.
9.   Bulun, S. E., Noble, L. S., Takayama, K. *et al.* (1997). 'Endocrine disorders associated with inappropriately high aromatase expression', *Journal of Steroid Biochemistry and Molecular Biology* 61(3-6):133-39
10.   Wilkin, T. J. and Voss, L. D. (2004). 'Metabolic syndrome: maladaptation to a modern world', *Journal of the Royal Society of Medicine* 97: 511-20
11.   Zhang, S. M., Lee, I., Manson, J. E. *et al.* (2007). 'Alcohol consumption and breast cancer risk in the women's health study', *American Journal of Epidemiology* 165(6): 667-76
12.   Maskarinec, G., Morimoto, Y., Takata, Y. *et al.* (2005). 'Alcohol and dietary fibre intakes affect circulating sex hormones among premenopausal women', *Public Health Nutrition* 9(7): 875-81
13.   Gunter, M. J., Hoover, D. R., Yu, H. *et al.* (2008). 'Insulin, insulin-like growth factor-I and risk of breast cancer in postmenopausal women', *Journal of the National Cancer Institute* 101(1): 48-60
14.   Key, T. J., Schatzkin, A., Willett, W. C., Allen, N. E., Spencer, E. A. and Travis, R. C. (2004). 'Diet, nutrition and the prevention of cancer', *Public Health Nutrition* (7)(1A): 187-200
15.   McTiernan, A., Tworoger, S. S., Ulrich, C. M. *et al.* (2004). 'Effect of exercise on serum estrogens in postmenopausal women. A 12-month randomized clinical trial', *Cancer Research* 64: 2923-28
16.   Campbell, K. L., Westerlind, K. C., Harber, V. J. *et al.* (2007). 'Effects of Aerobic Exercise Training on Estrogen Metabolism in Premenopausal Women: A Randomized Controlled Trial', *Cancer Epidemiology Biomarkers and Prevention* 16 (4): 731
17.   Colborn, T., Dumanoski, D. and Peterson Myers, J. (1996). *Our Stolen Future*. London: Abacus
18.   Ibid.
19.   The Medicines and Healthcare Products Regulatory Agency (MHRA) www.mhra.gov.uk *Hormone-replacement therapy: safety update. UK Public Assessment Report*. September 2007
20.   Drinking Water Inspectorate. www.dwi.gov.uk accessed September 2009

21. Colborn, Dumanoski and Peterson Myers, op cit.

22. Carlsen, E., Giwercman, A., Keiding, N., Skakkebaek, N. E. (1992). 'Evidence for decreasing quality of semen during past 50 years', *British Medical Journal* 305: 609-13

23. Wagner, M. and Oehlmann, J. (2009). 'Endocrine disruptors in bottled mineral water: total estrogenic burden and migration from plastic bottles', *Environmental Science and Pollution Research* 16(3): 278-86

24. Ben-Jonathan, N. and Steinmetz, R. (1998). 'Xenoestrogens: The emerging story of bisphenol A', *Trends in Endocrinology and Metabolism* 9(3): 124-28

25. Harvey, P. W. and Darbre, P. (2004). 'Endocrine disrupters and human health: Could oestrogenic chemicals in body care cosmetics adversely affect breast cancer incidence in women?', *Journal of Applied Toxicology* 24: 167-76

26. Darbre, P. and Harvey, P. W. (2008). 'Paraben esters: review of recent studies of endocrine toxicity, absorption, esterase and human exposure, and discussion of potential human health risks', *Journal of Applied Toxicology* 28(5): 561-78

27. McKinlay, R., Bella, J. N. B and Voulvoulis, N. (2008). 'Endocrine disrupting pesticides: implications for risk assessment', *Environment International* 34(2): 168-83

28. Carruba, G., Granata, O. M., Pala V. *et al.* (2006). 'A traditional Mediterranean diet decreases endogenous estrogens in healthy postmenopausal women', *Nutrition and Cancer* 56(2): 253-59

29. Ibid.

30. Cassidy, A. (2003). 'Potential risks and benefits of phytoestrogen-rich diets', *International Journal for Vitamin and Nutrition Research* 73(2): 120-26

31. Rice, S. and Whitehead, S. A. (2006). 'Phytoestrogens and breast cancer – promoters or protectors?', *Endocrine-Related Cancer* 13(4): 995-1015

32. Ibid.

33. Rowland, I., Faughnan, M., Hoey, L. *et al.* (2003). 'Bioavailability of phyto-oestrogens', *British Journal of Nutrition* 89 Supplement 1: S45-S58

34. Liu, J., Burdette, J. E., Xu, H. *et al.* (2001). 'Evaluation of
     estrogenic activity of plant extracts for the potential treatment
     of menopausal symptoms', *Journal of Agricultural and Food
     Chemistry* 49(5): 2472-79
35. He, Z., Chen, R. and Zhou, Y. (2009). 'Treatment for premenstrual
     syndrome with Vitex agnus castus: A prospective, randomized,
     multi-center placebo controlled study in China', *Maturitas* 63(1):
     99-103

SOLUTION 6

1.   Durrant-Peatfield, B. (2006) *Your Thyroid and How to Keep it
     Healthy.* London: Hammersmith Press
2.   Johnson, J. L. (2006). 'Diabetes control in thyroid disease',
     Diabetes Spectrum 19(3): 148
3.   Susheela, A. K., Bhatnagar, M., Vig, K. and Mondal, N. K. (2005).
     'Excess fluoride ingestion and thyroid derangements in children
     living in Delhi, India', *Fluoride* 38(2): 98-108
4.   Zimmermann, M., Jooste, P. L. and Pandav, C. (2008). 'Iodine-
     deficiency disorders', *The Lancet* 372(9645): 1251-62
5.   Garrow, J. S., James, W. P. T. and Ralph, A. (eds) (2000). *Human
     Nutrition and Dietetics.* London: Churchill Livingstone
6.   Vitti, P., Rago, T., Aghini-Lombardi, F. and Pinchera, A. (2001).
     'Iodine deficiency disorders in Europe', *Public Health Nutrition*
     4(2b): 529-35
7.   Ibid.
8.   Zimmermann, M. and Delange, F. (2004). 'Iodine supplementation
     of pregnant women in Europe: a review of recommendations',
     European Journal of Clinical Nutrition 58: 979-84
9.   Rayman, M., Sleeth, M., Walter, A. and Taylor, A. (2008). 'Iodine
     deficiency in UK women of child-bearing age', *Proceedings of the
     Nutrition Society* 67 (OCE8): E399
10. Ibid.
11. Lightowler, H. J. and Davies, G. J. (1998). 'Iodine intake and
     iodine deficiency in vegans as assessed by the duplicate-portion

technique and urinary iodine excretion', *British Journal of Nutrition* 80: 529-35

12. Kibirige, M. S., Hutchison, S., Owen, C. J. and Delves, H. (2004). 'Prevalence of maternal dietary iodine insufficiency in the north east of England: implications for the fetus', *Archives of Disease in Childhood Fetal and Neonatal Edition* 89(5): F436-F439

13. Henderson, L., Irving, K. and Gregory, J. (2003). *The national diet and nutrition survey: adults aged 19 to 64 years.* FSA and Department of Health

14. Fatourechi, V. (2009). 'Subclinical Hypothyroidism: An Update for Primary Care Physicians', *Mayo Clinic Proceedings* 84(1): 65-71

15. McDermott, M. T. and Ridgway, E. C. (2001). 'Subclinical hypothyroidism is mild thyroid failure and should be treated', *Journal of Clinical Endocrinology and Metabolism* 86(10): 4585-90

16. Fatourechi (2009) op cit.

17. McDermott and Ridgway (2001) op cit.

18. Ibid.

19. Ibid.

20. Ibid.

21. Fatourechi (2009) op cit.

22. Garrow, James and Ralph (2000) op cit.

23. Fontana, L., Klein, S., Holloszy, J. O. and Premachandra, B. N. (2006). 'Effect of long-term calorie restriction with adequate protein and micronutrients on thyroid hormones', *Journal of Clinical Endocrinology and Metabolism* 91(8): 3232-35

24. Fatourechi (2009) op cit.; McDermott and Ridgway (2001) op cit.

25. Rayman, M. P. (1997). 'Dietary selenium: Time to act', *British Medical Journal* 314: 387-88

26. Chrousos, G. P. (1997). 'Stressors, stress, and neuroendorcrine integration of the adaptive response'. The 1997 Hans Selye Memorial Lecture. National Institutes of Health, Bethesda.

SOLUTION 7

1. Edwards, C. A. and Parrett, A. M. (2002). 'Intestinal flora during

the first months of life: new perspectives', *British Journal of Nutrition* 88 (Suppl 1): S11-S18

2. Saavedra, J. M. and Tschernia, A. (2002). 'Human studies with probiotics and prebiotics: clinical implications', *British Journal of Nutrition* 87(Suppl.2): S241-S246

3. Edwards and Parrett (2002) op cit.

4. Sandek, A., Anker, S. D. and Haehling, S. V. (2009). 'The gut and intestinal bacteria in chronic heart failure', *Current Drug Metabolism* 10(1): 22-28(7)

5. British Nutrition Foundation. www.nutrition.org.uk accessed November 2009

6. Round, J. L. and Mazmaniam, S. K. (2009). 'The gut microbiota shapes intestinal immune responses during health and disease', *Nature Review/Immunology* 9: 313-23

7. Linskens, R. K., Huijsdens, X. W., Savelkoul, P. H. *et al.* (2001). 'The bacterial flora in inflammatory bowel disease: current insights in pathogenesis and the influence of antibiotics and probiotics', *Scandinavian Journal of Gastroenterology. Supplement* (234): 29-40

8. Round and Mazmaniam (2009) op cit.

9. Amin, O. M. (2002). 'Seasonal prevalence of intestinal parasites in the United States during 2000', *American Journal of Tropical Medicine and Hygiene* 66(6): 799-803

10. Santelmann, H. and McClaren Howard, J. (2005). 'Yeast metabolic products, yeast antigens and yeasts as possible triggers for irritable bowel syndrome', *European Journal of Gastroenterology and Hepatology* 17(1): 21-26

11. Ibid.

12. Fooks, L. J. and Gibson, G. R. (2002). 'Probiotics as modulators of the gut flora', *British Journal of Nutrition* 88 (Suppl 1): S39-S49

13. Boorom, K. F., Smith, H., Nimri, L. *et al.* (2008). 'Oh my aching gut: irritable bowel syndrome, Blastocystis, and asymptomatic infection', *Parasites and vectors,* 1: 40

14. Knowles, S. R., Nelson, E. A. and Palombo, E. A. (2008). 'Investigating the role of perceived stress on bacterial flora activity and salivary cortisol secretion: A possible mechanism underlying

susceptibility to illness', *Biological Psychology* 77(2): 132-37

15. Freestone, P. P. E., Sandrini, S. M., Haigh, R. D. and Lyte, M. (2008). 'Microbial endocrinology: how stress influences susceptibility to infection', *Trends in Microbiology* 16(2): 55-64

16. Fooks and Gibson (2002) op cit.

17. Woodmansey, E. J. (2007). 'Intestinal bacteria and ageing', *Journal of Applied Microbiology* 102: 1178-86

18. Ibid.

19. Bauer, E., Williams, B. A., Smidt, H. *et al.* (2006). 'Influence of dietary components on development of the microbiota in single-stomached species', *Nutrition Research Reviews* 19:63-78

20. Tuohy, K. M., Rouzaud, G. C. M., Brück, W. M. and Gibson, G. R. (2005). 'Modulation of the human gut microflora towards improved health using prebiotics – assessment of efficacy', *Current Pharmaceutical Design* 11: 75-90

21. Langlands, S. J., Hopkins, M. J., Coleman, N. and Cummings, J. H. (2004). 'Prebiotic carbohydrates modify the mucosa associated microflora of the human large bowel', *Gut* 53(11): 1610-16

22. Kruis, W., Forstmaier, G., Scheurlen, C. and Stellaard, F. (1991). 'Effect of diets low and high in refined sugars on gut transit, bile acid metabolism, and bacterial fermentation', *Gut* 32: 367-71

23. Ibid.

24. Abu-Elteen, K. H. (2005). 'The influence of dietary carbohydrates on in vitro adherence of four Candida species to human buccal epithelial cells', *Microbial Ecology in Health and Disease*, 17(3): 156-62

25. Johansson, N. L., Pavia, C. S. and Chiao, J. W. (2008). 'Growth inhibition of a spectrum of bacterial and fungal pathogens by sulforaphane, an isothiocyanate product found in broccoli and other cruciferous vegetables', *Planta Medica* 74(7): 747-50

26. Bauer, Williams, Smidt (2006) op cit.

27. Goldberg, M. J., Smith, J. W. and Nichols, R. L. (1977). 'Comparison of the fecal microflora of Seventh-Day Adventists with individuals consuming a general diet. Implications concerning colonic carcinoma', *Annals of Surgery* 186(1): 97-100

28. Bauer, Williams, Smidt (2006) op cit.
29. Tlaskalová-Hogenová, H., Stepánková, R., Hudcovic, T. *et al.* (2004). 'Commensal bacteria (normal microflora), mucosal immunity and chronic inflammatory and autoimmune diseases', *Immunology Letters* 15(93)(2-3): 97–108
30. Tuohy, Rouzaud, Brück and Gibson (2005), op cit.
31. Fooks and Gibson (2002) op cit.
32. Ibid.
33. Tuohy, Rouzaud, Brück and Gibson (2005), op cit.
34. Hébuterne, X. (2003). 'Gut changes attributed to ageing: effects on intestinal microflora', *Current Opinion in Clinical Nutrition and Metabolic Care* 6(1): 49-54
35. Woodmansey (2007) op cit.
36. Ibid.
37. Ibid.
38. Bauer, Williams, Smidt (2006) op cit.
39. Health Protection Agency (2008) 'Antimicrobial Resistance and Prescribing in England, Wales and Northern Ireland', London: Health Protection Agency
40. Soil Association. www.soilassociation.org accessed November 2009
41. Donaldson, L. (2009). '150 years of the annual report of the chief medical officer: On the state of public health, 2008', Department of Health
42. Ibid.
43. Murakami, M., Ohtake, T., Dorschner, R. A., *et al.* (2002). 'Cathelicidin Anti-Microbial Peptide Expression in Sweat, an Innate Defense System for the Skin', *Journal of Investigative Dermatology* 119: 1090–95
44. Schittek, B., Paulmann, M., Senyürek, I. and Steffen, H. (2008). 'The role of antimicrobial peptides in human skin and in skin infectious diseases', *Infectious Disorders – Drug Targets* 8(3): 135-43
45. Pivarcsi, A., Nagy, I. and Kemeny, L. (2005) 'Innate immunity in the skin: How keratinocytes fight against pathogens. *Current Immunology Reviews*, 1(1):29-42(14).

SOLUTION 8

1. Purohit, V., Bode, J. C., Bode, C. *et al.* (2008). 'Alcohol, intestinal bacterial growth, intestinal permeability to endotoxin, and medical consequences', *Alcohol* 42(5): 349-61
2. Clayburgh, D. R., Shen, L. and Turner, J. R. (2004). 'A porous defense: the leaky epithelial barrier in intestinal disease', *Laboratory Investigation* 84: 282-91
3. Dunlop, S. P., Hebden, J. and Campbell, E. *et al.* (2006). 'Abnormal Intestinal Permeability in Subgroups of Diarrhea-Predominant Irritable Bowel Syndromes', *The American Journal of Gastroenterology* 101(6): 1288-94
4. Ventura, M. T., Polimeno, L. and Amoruso, A. C. *et al.* (2006). 'Intestinal permeability in patients with adverse reactions to food', *Digestive and Liver Disease* 38(10): 732-36
5. Hijazi, Z., Molla, A. M., and Al Habashi, H. (2004). 'Intestinal permeability is increased in bronchial asthma', *Archives of Disease in Childhood* 89: 227-29
6. Camilleri, M. and Gorman H. (2007). 'Intestinal permeability and irritable bowel syndrome', *Neurogastroenterology and Motility* 19: 545-52
7. Spiller, R. and Campbell, E. (2006). 'Post-infectious irritable bowel syndrome', *Current Opinion in Gastroenterology,* 22(1): 13-17
8. Arrieta, M. C., Bistritz, L. and Meddings, J. B. (2006). 'Alterations in intestinal permeability', *Gut* 55(10): 1512-20
9. DeMeo, M. T., Mutlu, E. A., Keshavarzian, A. and Tobin, M. C. (2002). 'Intestinal permeation and gastrointestinal disease', *Journal of Clinical Gastroenterology* 34(4): 385-96
10. Laukoetter, M., Porfirio, N. and Nusrat, A. (2008). 'Role of the intestinal barrier in inflammatory bowel disease', *World Journal of Gastroenterology* 14(3): 401-407
11. Clayburgh, Shen and Turner (2004) op cit.
12. Arrieta, Bistritz and Meddings (2006) op cit.
13. DeMeo, Mutlu, Keshavarzian and Tobin (2002) op cit.
14. Ibid.

15. Ibid.
16. Ibid.
17. Ibid.
18. Maes, M., Kubera, M. and Leunis, J.C. (2008). 'The gut–brain barrier in major depression: Intestinal mucosal dysfunction with an increased translocation of LPS from gram negative enterobacteria (leaky gut) plays a role in the inflammatory pathophysiology of depression', *Neuroendocrinology Letters* 29(1): 117-24
19. Maes, M., Coucke, F. and Leunis, J.C. (2007). 'Normalization of the increased translocation of endotoxin from gram negative enterobacteria (leaky gut) is accompanied by a remission of chronic fatigue syndrome', *Neuroendocrinology Letters* 28(6): 739-44
20. Venket Rao, A., Bested, A. C., Beaulne, T. M. (2009). 'A randomized, double-blind, placebo-controlled pilot study of a probiotic in emotional symptoms of chronic fatigue syndrome', *Gut Pathogens* 1: 6
21. Arrieta, Bistritz and Meddings (2006) op cit.
22. Bosi, E., Molteni, L. and Radaelli, M. G. *et al*. (2006). 'Increased intestinal permeability precedes clinical onset of type 1 diabetes', *Diabetologia* 49(12): 2824-27
23. Rosenfeldt, V., Benfeldt, E., Valerius, N. *et al*. (2004). 'Effect of probiotics on gastrointestinal symptoms and small intestinal permeability in children with atopic dermatitis', *The Journal of Pediatrics* 145(5): 612-16
24. Orlando, A., Renna, S., Perricone, G. and Cottone, M. (2009). 'Gastrointestinal lesions associated with spondyloarthropathies', *World Journal of Gastroenterology* 15(20): 2443-48
25. Arrieta, Bistritz and Meddings (2006) op cit.
26. Orlando, Renna, Perricone and Cottone (2009) op cit.
27. DeMeo, Mutlu, Keshavarzian and Tobin (2002) op cit.
28. Penalva, J. C., Martínez, J. and Laveda, R. *et al*. (2004). 'A study of intestinal permeability in relation to the inflammatory response and plasma endocab IgM levels in patients with acute pancreatitis', *Journal of Clinical Gastroenterology* 38(6): 512-17

29. Arrieta, Bistritz and Meddings (2006) op cit.
30. Spiller, R. C., Jenkins, D. and Thornley, J. P. (2000). 'Increased rectal mucosal enteroendocrine cells, T lymphocytes, and increased gut permeability following acute Campylobacter enteritis and in post-dysenteric irritable bowel syndrome', *Gut* 47: 804-11
31. Spiller and Campbell (2006) op cit.
32. Orlando, Renna, Perricone and Cottone (2009) op cit.
33. Soderholm, J. D. and Perdue, M. H. (2001). 'Stress and the gastrointestinal tract II. Stress and intestinal barrier function', *American Journal of Physiology – Gastrointestinal and Liver Physiology* 280: G7-G13
34. Rao, R. K., Polk, D. B., Seth, A. and Yan, F. (2009). 'Probiotics the good neighbor: Guarding the gut mucosal barrier', *American Journal of Infectious Diseases* 5(3): 195-99
35. Laukoetter, Porfirio and Nusrat (2008) op cit.
36. Rao, Polk, Seth and Yan (2009) op cit.
37. Rosenfeldt, Benfeldt, Valerius *et al.* (2004) op cit
38. DeMeo, Mutlu, Keshavarzian and Tobin (2002) op cit.
39. Garcia Vilela, E., De Lourdes De Abreu Ferrari, M., Oswaldo Da Gama Torres, H. *et al.* (2008). 'Influence of Saccharomyces boulardii on the intestinal permeability of patients with Crohn's disease in remission', *Scandinavian Journal of Gastroenterology* 43(7): 842-48
40. Purohit, Bode *et al.* (2008) op cit.
41. Hond, E. D., Peeters, M., Hiele, M. *et al.* (1999). 'Effect of glutamine on the intestinal permeability changes induced by indomethacin in humans', *Alimentary Pharmacology and Therapeutics* 13(5): 679-85
42. De-Souza, D. A. and Greene, L. J. (2005). 'Intestinal permeability and systemic infections in critically ill patients: Effect of glutamine', *Critical Care Medicine* 33(5): 1125-35
43. Ibid.
44. Langmead, L., Makins, R. J. and Rampton, D. S. (2004). 'Anti-inflammatory effect of aloe vera gel in human colorectal mucosa in vitro. *Alimentary Pharmacology and Therapeutics,* 19(5): 521-27

45. Langmead, L., Feakins, R. M. and Goldthorpe, S. *et al.* (2004). 'Randomized, double-blind, placebo-controlled trial of oral aloe vera gel for active ulcerative colitis', *Alimentary Pharmacology and Therapeutics* 19(7): 739-47

46. Purohit, Bode *et al.* (2008) op cit.

47. Ibid.

Index

Hay House Titles of Related Interest

Health Bliss,
by Susan Smith Jones

L Is for Labels,
by Amanda Ursell

The PCOS Protection Plan,
by Colette Harris and Theresa Cheung

PCOS and Your Fertility,
by Colette Harris and Theresa Cheung

Spent?,
by Frank Lipman

Waist Disposal,
by Dr John Briffa

What Are You Really Eating?,
by Amanda Ursell

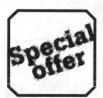

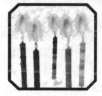

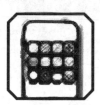
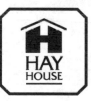

ABOUT THE AUTHOR

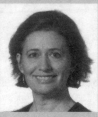

Maria Cross studied nutritional therapy at the Institute for Optimum Nutrition in London, graduating in 1994. Since then she has helped thousands of people overcome a wide range of common symptoms. Recognizing that individuals live in societies and environments that impact on their health and wellbeing, she developed an interest in public health and went on to graduate with an MSc in Public Health Food and Nutrition. She joined the University of Westminster in 2000 where she was a lecturer and clinic tutor on the first nutritional therapy degree course in the country. Maria has made regular contributions to health magazines, and her first co-authored book, *Nutrition in Institutions*, was published in 2009.

Maria is a member of the British Association for Applied Nutrition and Nutritional Therapy (BANT) and the Guild of Health Writers. She lives with her husband in Hertfordshire.

www.mariacross.co.uk